£30.00

Cicely Saunders.
1996.

THERAPY ABATEMENT, AUTONOMY AND FUTILITY

To Storm, Daisy and Baskie

Therapy Abatement, Autonomy and Futility

Ethical Decisions at the Edge of Life

DAVID LAMB

Avebury
Aldershot • Brookfield USA • Hong Kong • Singapore • Sydney

© D. Lamb 1995

All rights reserved. No part of this publication may be reproduced, stored in a retrieval system, or transmitted in any form or by any means, electronic, mechanical, photocopying, recording or otherwise without the prior permission of the publisher.

Published by
Avebury
Ashgate Publishing Limited
Gower House
Croft Road
Aldershot
Hants GU11 3HR
England

Ashgate Publishing Company
Old Post Road
Brookfield
Vermont 05036
USA

British Library Cataloguing in Publication Data

Lamb, David
   Therapy Abatement, Autonomy and Futility:
   Ethical Decisions at the Edge of Life
   I. Title
   174.2

ISBN 1 85972 202 4

Library of Congress Catalog Card Number: 95-78193

Printed and bound in Great Britain by
Ipswich Book Co. Ltd., Ipswich, Suffolk

Contents

Acknowledgements		vi
Chapter I	Introduction: Is Philosophy Relevant to Medical Decision Making?	1
Chapter II	Therapy Abatement and Euthanasia	17
Chapter III	Advance Directives and Living Wills	38
Chapter IV	'Do Not Attempt to Resuscitate' Orders	62
Chapter V	Futile Therapy	74
Chapter VI	Nutrition and Hydration	91
Chapter VII	Therapy Abatement When Treatment is Expensive	101
Chapter VIII	Autonomous Refusal	112
Chapter IX	Autonomy and Surrogacy	128
Bibliography		137
Index		144

Acknowledgements

Quite a number of people have contributed in various ways to the completion of this manuscript. I would like to thank Kim Bevington for valuable secretarial help throughout the project, especially during the latter stages, and also Wendy Howat and Pat Rarity. Many thanks also to Susan Easton and Doris Schroeder who made helpful criticism on earlier drafts of the book. As various chapters have been offered in university courses and conferences I would like to thank those who participated in them for forcing me to clarify some of the ideas expressed here. In particular, thanks to the students of the Applied Ethics course during my last year as a lecturer at the University of Manchester; staff and postgraduates in the Department of Biomedical Science and Bioethics, University of Birmingham; participants at the Conference on Euthanasia held at the University of Kent, March, 1995, and a word of special thanks for the robust criticism from members of the Swindon Philosophical Society who, for some inexplicable reason, continue to reinvite me to lecture on topics featured in this book. The cost for the preparation of this manuscript was met by an award from the University Research Support Fund: Small Grants, at the University of Manchester. For this I am most grateful.

D. Lamb

I Introduction: Is Philosophy Relevant to Medical Decision Making?

In recent years there has been a sustained backlash against applied ethics, particularly in the field of medicine, from certain members of the medical profession and traditional philosophers who have expressed doubts concerning the role of applied ethics. Some critics have dismissed applied ethics as a ruse to obtain teaching posts. Others view the applied ethicist as a person who has given up on the really difficult problem of 'mainstream' philosophy. On the other hand it is also said that applied ethics offers an escape from a profession obsessed by unreal puzzles, trivia and irrelevant arguments. The question of philosophy's contribution to moral decision-making in medicine deserves to be addressed directly.

Anne Maclean (1993) has argued that bioethicists and applied ethicists are incapable of making any contribution to health-care and that they lack any special expertise which can be applied to ethical problems in medicine. Maclean's argument could be regarded as a development of Wittgenstein's notorious slogan that 'philosophy leaves everything as it is', which reflected his belief that philosophy was not a genuine subject, could make no claims to advance knowledge, and resulted from various forms of linguistic confusion. Like Wittgenstein, Maclean dismisses many of the arguments of contemporary bioethicists - whom she wrongly identifies as utilitarians of one sort or another - in favour of appeals to 'what ordinary people believe', or 'what most of us think' or 'what strikes us'. Such appeals to ordinary commonsense intuition are useful counter-measures to some of the wilder proposals of utilitarian and consequentialist doctrines. But the declaration that philosophy is unfit to address some of the major moral issues of our time is clearly contestable. Bad philosophy can be corrected by good philosophy which can demonstrate why the former was unfit to address the problems. But a philosophy which confesses its own ineptitude has abandoned the right to pass comment and judgement on the philosophy of others. What really happens when philosophers withdraw from moral discourse is that others - who may or may not describe themselves as philosophers - continue to address the problems. Now it may be, as Maclean argues, that some approaches to philosophy make illicit claims regarding their access to truth and reason. But arguments designed to demonstrate the weaknesses and inadequacies of some standpoints cannot be extended to the entire scope of philosophical inquiry.

Nevertheless, Maclean is partly correct in her criticism of the claim that philosophers possess a special expertise and when she insists that there is not *one* rational answer to the moral problems in medicine. Philosophers simply do not possess any special skills or theories which can be produced to resolve any of life's dilemmas. But this is not to concede the case that philosophy has something to contribute to other disciplines. There is an important contribution that philosophers can make to medicine - and other disciplines too - which Maclean herself outlines when she refers to the questions that can be raised in response to a proposed action: 'Why is it a moral issue at all for us? How does it connect up with other issues? What values does it put at stake? What are the implications of deciding it in a particular way, or of arguing in a particular way?' (Maclean 1993:202)

There are two very elementary approaches to moral philosophy which can tell us about the nature of philosophical inquiry and indicate why it is felt to be inappropriate when applied to professional life. First, there is an approach which consists of testing a proposed principle against our ordinary intuitions concerning right or wrong. For example, someone might propose a certain form of punishment as a deterrent to other potential wrong-doers, but is then confronted with an objection that this particular proposal could lead to a situation where the innocent could be punished. In this way a dilemma is introduced between the moral belief that wrong-doers should be deterred and the belief that the innocent should not be punished. Attempts to resolve this dilemma may involve reflection on our moral beliefs regarding punishment and in the course of the inquiry one may even revise one's original intuitions. A second approach to moral philosophy could involve a demonstration of unforeseen or unintended consequences of a set of beliefs. This method was used by Socrates. Some unwitting Greek would claim that truth-telling was one of the highest virtues and Socrates would then manufacture examples where truth-telling would bring about evil. The Socratic objective was not to encourage a community of liars, but to lead his protagonist into further reflection on the complexities surrounding our notions of truth and virtue.

These approaches are generally successful in introducing philosophy students to the discipline. They will have been told that everyday intuitions can be challenged and they are prepared for bizarre challenges to well-established principles concerning good conduct. But specialists in other disciplines may not take kindly to an approach which seemingly trivialises and easily dismisses beliefs and moral principles that have evolved, consolidated, and stood the test of time. For example, critical-care staff work within a framework of professional values and guidelines for patient care that have been well-established, published in journals, taught to students, criticised and occasionally revised. These guidelines may need further revision in the light of new developments in the provision of care. But these values are deeply imbedded in the practice of critical-care and will not be easily suspended in response to a philosopher's seemingly playful introduction of bizarre situations where well-meaning guidelines break down. The most likely response of the professional will be the dismissal of philosophy as inappropriate. Some of the reasons why philosophy is considered to be inappropriate to medical decision-making will now be considered.

Is Applied Ethics Irrelevant?

Robert Zussman (1992:2) has criticised recent medical ethics because it has 'consistently ignored the social context in which medical decisions are made', stressing formal procedures for obtaining a patient's consent to treatment and thus ignoring the social forces that shape peoples' values. There is, of course, a reverse side to this complaint: the success of applied ethics has been very much bound up with widespread recourse throughout contemporary society to formal procedures. This can be seen in recent criticism of advance directives, or living wills, which cannot substitute for an interactive relationship between carer and patient.

Failure to consider the wider context in which medical decisions are taken leads to the complaint that a great deal of philosophical argument, examples and counter-examples, assumes a kind of static existence of the problems. This is reinforced by conventions in the teaching of philosophy, supported by tacit consent which rule out certain data as irrelevant. For example, when presenting well-worn dilemmas it is considered inappropriate to confuse the argument with too much data. This is particularly notorious in discussions of ethical problems generated out of the 'acts and omissions' distinction where it is customary only to present a limited amount of information about the case. Just enough, perhaps, to establish that the patient will die if one acts in a certain way and will also die if one fails to act. A discussion on the patient's case history, or on other comparable cases, would be beside the point. The point of limiting factual information is that the student can recognize the 'relevant' theoretical position without being led astray by 'irrelevant' case histories and other 'extraneous details'. Yet it may be precisely these other details which, when subjected to moral scrutiny, can lead to a greater understanding of the problem and the underlying assumptions of those involved in it, and eventual steps towards a solution or reconciliation. Human preferences and needs are also assumed to be static by many teachers of philosophy. Thus issues like euthanasia can be discussed where the moral weight attributed to faculties such as consciousness and cognitive skills remains constant. But in the real world interests and needs are constantly changing and evolving. Patients may come to tolerate illness, nurses may lose interest in some patients and relatives completely contradict earlier requests.

Philosophy as a Means of Clarification

Some philosophers have insisted that philosophy does not provide a technique for solving moral problems but instead the expertise they can offer consists in various methods of clarifying the issues. But if this is the case then how does it clarify? The usual answer is that clarification is somehow obtained by a process of relating conflicting claims about good conduct to familiar ethical theories. When this is done the philosophically minded can then continue with the evaluation of the various conflicting arguments underlying ethical theories thus leaving an overall impression that instead of clarifying the issues, the philosopher has merely retreated into a debate on theoretical abstractions.

Clarification may be achieved through conceptual analysis. But there are limits to this approach. For example, the substitution of a moral argument for a definition of a concept does not dispel serious doubts about the morality of continuing or terminating a pregnancy or not providing or withholding a form of life-prolonging therapy. One of the most harmful legacies of recent philosophy has been attempts to provide definitions of personhood as a yardstick for moral relevance. Appeals to loss of personhood have been advanced in arguments designed to extend the criteria for diagnosing brain death to persistent vegetative state (PVS) patients who, whilst displaying no conscious activity are alive insofar as they have a functioning brainstem. Such arguments are advanced in apparent ignorance of the facts that (a) diagnosis of the PVS is indeterminate and (b) we are far from reaching a social consensus concerning personhood or its loss. (Lamb, 1992)

Diversionary Ethics

Applied ethics can also be employed in a diversionary manner: a philosopher hired to discuss the allocation of scarce resources can divert attention from the very real problem that society and its government is unwilling to provide adequate funds for those who need them. This can be seen on a national scale: the Government initiates a policy of cuts in health-care expenditure and philosophers appear on the media with proposals and criteria for a just system for allocating the ever shrinking supply. At the very least a philosopher should pose questions concerning the scarcity assumption which underpins every rationing proposal.

Applied ethics may also be trivialised to the point where it is seen as nothing more than an opportunity to let off steam. An ethicist can be employed in a hospital and become a useful catharsis for nurses and other personnel with a grievance to direct their anger and frustration. Controversial issues can be sidetracked by remit to a committee ran by an applied ethicist where angry words can be spoken and heard by an academic who possesses no executive authority. Far from digging out the *real* problems, ethical analysis so frequently sidetracks legitimate complaints. In this respect there is a very real danger that ethical discourse will come to function as a diversion from questions of public accountability.

Engineering Ethics

Philosophers, we have noted, are frequently criticised for conducting arguments which appear inappropriate to lay persons and professionals in other disciplines. Sometimes this criticism is justified. But in another sense dissatisfaction with philosophy's role in medical decision-making is not due to its inappropriateness but is very much bound up with the medical community's expectations of philosophy, which in turn is also bound up with some of the aims and objectives of philosophers themselves. Arthur Caplan (1992:xii) sees fundamental problems in what he describes as 'engineering ethics' or 'universal foundationalism', which seeks 'unassailable foundations for normative statements and presumes the same theory which is used to shed light on one domain of morality will work equally well in another direction'. This view can be held by philosophers and professionals in other disciplines who expect the philosopher to produce a set of unshakeable moral foundations for their discipline. Foundationalists believe that only one moral theory can underpin a moral outlook and consequently see applied ethics as a second-order discipline which awaits the perfection or near perfection of the foundational theory. Then the theory can be *applied* to the moral problems of the day, irrespective of changes in scientific theory, medical research or major cultural developments. The real business of philosophy, argues the foundationalist, is to establish and test the underpinning theory. Such concerns can be irritating to the scientist and medical practitioner. To give an example: I once heard a philosopher addressing a problem in the philosophy of mind and she produced a fictitious example of piecing a large collection of neurones together to make a complete brain, but then she forestalled any scientific objections with references to 'future developments in the neurosciences with blah-de-blah-de-blah'! In this way the audience were directed towards the supposedly *real* philosophical questions and were not distracted by considerations whether they had any plausibility or practical relevance. I have not produced this example in order to criticise a way of doing philosophy, but to show the limits of this way of doing applied philosophy.

Foundationalism in ethics is marred by its unhistorical formalistic character and in this respect it resembles logical positivism in the philosophy of science. As Caplan points out, ethical foundationalists believe that ethics must be grounded upon a valid theory, based on a set of axioms or unchallengeable truths. The principles and rules of the theory are deduced from the axioms and the objective is that other foundationalist philosophers will test the theory by finding (usually fictitious) moral problems which are inconsistent with one of the claims deduced from the principles or axioms. Students can be introduced to this approach by being asked questions which limit the parameters of ethical discourse to challenges to foundational theories: for example, how would a utilitarian deal with proposals to withdraw nutrition and hydration from patients who are in a PVS? Would a version of hedonistic or preference utilitarianism be more successful in dealing with the problem? Can Kantian principles justify surrogate decision-making on behalf of decisionally incapacitated patients? This method of simplifying and idealising the nature and structure of moral problems is unhelpful to doctors, nurses, patient communities and relatives who may well be wrestling with urgent moral problems concerning therapy options for terminally ill patients and are not idly awaiting the confirmation of some foundational theory.

There is an assumption in much applied philosophy in the engineering tradition that ethical problems are self-evident and await the application of an appropriate theory to resolve them. Put in rather simplistic terms this reflects the belief that a health-care professional encounters a moral problem and then presents it to a philosopher who can run it through a few moral theories and come up with a piece of advice. On these terms there is no essential difference between encountering a moral problem in a philosophy examination and a hospital ward. This approach to applied philosophy shares some similarities with the model of a primary clinical examination. The doctor encounters a problem described by the patient and applies her knowledge to the data and offers appropriate advice. But the difference is that the moral problem is taken at face value whereas, to emulate the clinician, the philosopher should feel free to re-describe the problem, evaluate its component parts, and above all be prepared to transcend the range of solutions given initially with the problem. Thus, as in a clinical examination, the patient's description and perceived dilemmas, may have to be reorganised and a new set of problems may have to be introduced in the light of philosophical reflection. The engineering approach also fails to recognise that the ethicist, like the doctor, makes assumptions, and consequently the exponent of the engineering approach portrays ethical dilemmas as problems supplied by the client. This, too, is part of the legacy of positivism's belief that an investigator is strictly limited by the object.

Caplan (1992) critically examines three components of engineering ethics which have been offered to medical practice: conceptual analysis, the application of theories to problems, and the neutrality and objectivity of philosophical thinking. 1) Conceptual analysis assists with inquiries into the meaning of words, detection of logical fallacies, identification of confusion, and seeks to establish canons of sound argumentation. 2) Philosophers claim to be able to bring a body of specialist knowledge of ethical theories to the moral problems of medicine. The philosopher can show how certain moral theories can be applied to problems, just as the engineer draws from theories in physics to solve problems with a heating system. 3) Philosophy encourages neutrality and objectivity; philosophers are impartial observers, whose advice is uncluttered by either emotional or specialist interests.

How successful is the engineering model? Some success can be claimed with reference to the numbers of philosophers who have been influential in the formulation of health policy, chairing commissions, drafting regulations and contributing to the work of ethics committees. Philosophers have also been involved in the drafting of codes of ethics as more professional groups become aware of dilemmas and the need for codes of conduct. These activities seemingly suggest that there is an expertise to be applied by philosophers on many areas of professional conduct. But the model has rather limited success in the teaching of ethics to professional health-care workers. On the positive side, it can be said that quite a number of medical personnel have been attracted to philosophy and have gone on to complete Ph.D.'s in the subject, but more frequently students attending philosophy courses - as do a very large percentage of philosophy undergraduates - find the philosophy boring and irrelevant. Of course the philosophers can simply retort that a large percentage of their classes do not really appreciate philosophy, and their dissatisfaction is but an expression of their confused expectations. But this retort ignores the frustration felt by many health-care workers, having presented a specific case to a philosopher and obtained nothing more than a logic chopping discussion, with questions being answered by more evasive questions.

This dissatisfaction could be seen to be a direct result of the threefold promise of the engineering model: 1) Conceptual analysis, so it would seem, leads only to further analysis. 2) The claim that philosophers bring specialist knowledge of ethical theories is countered by the complaint that the theories are either too abstract or too fictitious, having little application in the real world. 3) The alleged neutrality of philosophy is even more irritating to professional health-care workers. Opponents in a fiercely fought debate are either irritated by the philosopher who 'sits on the fence', or they interpret the alleged neutrality as tacit support for the other side. It does not take long to discover that the impartial philosopher is easily manipulated into being a supporter for the more powerful interest groups. For example, from the administration's point of view an impartial academic is much more compliant than a strongly committed representative of a patient's organization. A few impartial academics on the relevant committees can effectively neutralize opposition to the administration's objectives. Institutions which adopt well-grounded, consistent and logically water-tight ethics codes, which have been endorsed by committee philosophers, can bypass local and national negotiating machinery to the disadvantage of employees.

The 'engineering model' is suggestive of a division of labour, whereby the non-professional (or expert in some other discipline than philosophy) encounters a moral problem and hands it over to be resolved by the philosopher who applies a body of well-confirmed ethical theory. James M. Brown has argued that this appeal to the division of labour is misguided: it is 'undesirable for non-philosophers such as doctors to have complete control of identification and characterization of problems to be solved' (Brown 1987:82). Moreover, as he points out, there is no body of well-grounded theory. There is also an important feature of morality which conflicts with the division of labour model: it is not always the case that a moral problem is recognized as a problem by the agents concerned. Normal routine behaviour may contain moral problems which are unrecognized by the agents concerned, and remain so until some irritating Socratic draws attention to them.

The diversification model of applied philosophy has also been criticised by Geoffrey Hunt who rejects the assumption, held by many teachers of applied philosophy, that the task of the philosopher is to search for and then deliver the right method of resolving ethical problems. Hunt (1994:4) is critical of the way many teachers of ethics courses for nurses 'appear convinced that a heavy dose of theories and principles carrying labels like "deontology or utilitarianism", "beneficence", "non-maleficence", "autonomy", "quality or sanctity of life" will fill the moral void in our health-care system'. For Hunt, part of the problem with applied ethics in the context of health-care is bound up with its imitation of the 'technocratic and curative approach to health', (*ibid*:4) and the related search for the 'technically right procedure or method for dealing with "ethical decisions"'. This approach suggests that health-care workers live in some kind of moral vacuum with no idea how to resolve their dilemmas. Yet as Hunt (*ibid*:5) points out: 'everyone knows that student nurses do *already* have the responses of honesty, promise-keeping, respect for others, privacy, self-esteem, and do understand these concepts'. In contrast Hunt (*ibid*:5) stresses exploration, involving 'free examination' of 'the conditions which create disparities between what their ordinary moral sense tells them and what they are expected to do without question'. Thus one of the key roles for applied philosophy is that of questioning institutional procedures and other obstacles that prevent people from acting in ways that they know to be right.

The Separation of Theory from Practice

A frequent complaint with philosophy is that philosophers have departed from the Aristotelian tradition of maintaining a unity between theory and practice. This view is developed by Gordon Dunstan (1995:3) who complains that much of applied philosophy is purely formal:

> Too much of it is word-play: a departmental game in which medical issues are batted like shuttlecocks from side to side, not for advancement of good medical practice, but to exercise or demonstrate skills in argument. Slogans are devised and canonised.... 'Autonomy' is exalted into an absolute claim, over-riding other legitimate claims. 'Rights' are multiplied, assumed or attributed where they do not exist, replacing the language of duties, which oblige even when there are no rights. These are the marks of the 'ethicists' in much of contemporary writing. They are not characteristic of competent philosophy, any more than the citing of Biblical or Vatican texts as conclusive against reason and moral experience is characteristic of moral philosophy.

According to Dunstan, when properly understood, expertise in philosophy is not divorced from practice and should not be employed to replace or undermine the moral decision-making of health-care professionals. Whatever expertise a philosopher may possess, in practical contexts the doctors are the moral agents whose 'duties and decisions at every stage relate to and are inseparable from the expertise required and exercised at every step. No philosopher, no "bioethicist", can or may usurp them. No true philosopher would wish to do so.' (Dunstan, 1995:5) It may seem trite to speak of doctors as moral agents. But emphasis on the contractual aspect of the doctor-patient relationship, the promotion of autonomy as a means of choosing commodities, suggests that doctors are mere suppliers of technical goods which a rational moral agent may either purchase or leave on the shelf.

What Can Philosophy Offer?

Having listed the complaints against applied philosophy, one might be forgiven in thinking that it should be discarded and that the philosopher has nothing to offer that could not be produced by any reasonably educated person. Most people have a clear sense of right and wrong and many institutions in a democratic society respect the individual's personal conscience. What is so special about philosophers that gives them authority to make special pronouncements about morality and virtue? If, as it is argued, they have no special expertise, do they possess moral authority? The idea that philosophers possess a degree of moral authority is largely resisted by philosophers despite Plato's claim in the *Republic* that autocratic government should be in the hands of philosophers. J.L. Gorman (1987) makes a relevant point when he draws attention to the two lessons of analytic philosophy: 'philosophers have no moral authority' and 'nobody else has moral authority'. Analytic philosophers see their inquiry as a form of second order work, and accordingly argue philosophy cannot directly address moral problems. But aside from this rather curious view of philosophy the idea of moral authority is not such a problem: at least two professions other than philosophy exercise it; law and politics. The philosopher with a burning desire to become a moral authority should be recommended to take Plato's advice and enter one of these professions. In some respects the denial of moral authority by philosophers is partly due to a belief in egalitarian values and partly due to a form of humility which finds expression in the work of many English philosophers. But to say that someone who is intellectually immersed in the ideas of the great figures in the history of moral philosophy has no moral authority is clearly absurd. An authority on Plato, or Aristotle, or Kant is, to a great extent, an authority on their moral wisdom. But at a minimal level, the authority exercised by philosophers is derived from the honesty, validity and relevance of their arguments. They ought to be skilled at presenting moral arguments and if they are they possess authority. Insofar as applied philosophy brings knowledge of the great intellectual traditions to a problem, moral authority is measured by the ability to apply them in a relevant and fruitful manner.

When pressed most philosophers would say that any claims to authority rests on a mixture of the following: an ability to reason well, avoid errors in argument and recognise them in the arguments of others. This is surely valuable but it is not enough; as we have argued, there has to be a subject-matter and philosophers must have some knowledge of it and respect for it. The great philosophers of the past were experts in some field other than logic. Aristotle was an expert in biology and Descartes was an expert in mathematics and the physical sciences. A reasonable knowledge of the ideas of the great philosophers is of positive value to everyone and an awareness of moral theories, their strengths and weaknesses, is a powerful prophylactic against the errors of personal conviction and emotional reaction. But to this we must add a requirement to be well informed about the relevant facts. This in turn requires some philosophical reflection on the actual discipline and respect for the facts and theoretical certainties which should not be dismissed with appeals to fictitious logical possibilities. It must also be acknowledged that ethical problems are not simply generated by the facts, but are generated by a combination of long-standing ethical beliefs and facts whose significance is subject to reinterpretation. The philosopher must possess a familiarity with the context in which certain facts become significant. Why, for example, do facts about the administration of artificial nutrition and hydration, have an ethical significance which transcends discussion about an organism's requirement for energy resources? Once engaged in the actual practices of a discipline the philosopher can make a meaningful contribution which need not be dismissed as an irrelevant exercise in logic chopping.

So what is the difference between the moral philosopher and the intelligent practitioner? There may not be one, as the latter may very well be engaged in a philosophical approach to the discipline. But frequently the philosophical contribution will not be in terms of the solution to a presented problem; the philosopher may draw attention to moral problems which no one had actually identified as problems. Thus much of applied philosophy - perhaps the most interesting part - lies, not in the search for an application of the best theory but in the identification of problems, rearranging them and recognising that the facts which are presented by doctors and nurses as constitutive of a moral dilemma may have to be re-arranged.

In some respects the philosopher can play a role similar to an innovator in a given discipline. The innovator may introduce new problems and solutions which lead to a questioning of traditional practices and a possible re-evaluation of their merits. Throughout history social groups have unquestioningly held beliefs which have later been subject to criticism and re-evaluation before being either discarded or reinforced. Assumptions concerning the sanctity of life have been held unquestioningly, discarded by some people and reinforced by others after reflection. The philosopher-innovator must tread carefully when examining deeply-held beliefs and avoid giving an impression that they are being lightly discarded. For this reason it is important that the philosopher, like the innovator, is aware of the facts and is sympathetic to problems actually encountered within the discipline under examination. Medicine today encounters deeply held assumptions regarding the status of the doctor as a moral agent, the importance of patient autonomy, as well as assumptions underpinning the two moral panics of our time; fear about over-treatment at the end of life, and threats concerning the distribution of scarce medical resources. Many of these assumptions will be related to values concerning what is believed to be an acceptable quality of life. A philosophical examination of these assumptions might involve posing questions like 'why do we regard this as a valuable objective?' 'Why do we continue to do things this way?' 'Do we have good reasons for continuing?' Good reasons might be provided but still remain within a framework of values that is questionable. Thus, for example, a doctor might propose moderately debilitating but nevertheless disfiguring surgery, as she has consistently done, with reference to a predictable increase in life-expectancy. This, she says, is why she will continue to do things this way, and the evidence of increased rates of life expectancy gives her a good reason for continuing. But her ethical framework could be questioned on the grounds that she has placed a greater value on the quantity of life over the quality of life and that given an autonomous choice her patient might well opt for the likelihood of a shorter life without disfigurement. In the event of a moral contest between the two positions there will be philosophical reflection on the notion of 'a good reason' and further reflection on the agency responsible for the decision. How much authority should the doctor wield and how much is the decision to rest with the autonomous patient? In the course of the inquiry attention will focus on the concept of 'benefit', 'autonomy', 'quality of life' and the moral status of the doctor.

Beyond these considerations there is the general perception that philosophers can relate particular moral problems to the big questions of life: what is truth, justice and freedom, and what does it mean to speak of the good life? There was a time when philosophers addressed serious issues, posing questions concerning how language can mean anything, which is a very big question. People expect big, or deep questions from philosophers and a hint at how deep a question is would be a useful contribution from philosophy.

It is not an objective here to provide new foundations for moral theory, although that certainly could be an intellectually stimulating task for philosophers to engage in. My objective, however, is to develop an old and familiar aspect of philosophy which involves raising questions, exposing hidden assumptions, planting seeds of doubt where certainty once ruled, and retaining the philosopher's freedom to explore problems and to restructure and manipulate the framework of any debate.

There is plenty of work for philosophers to undertake. One of the many contributions we can make is the task of separating different moral issues which frequently conflict and prevent the agent from pursuing ethically desirable goals. For example, many doctors may have strong ethical objections to either active or passive euthanasia, but have an equal moral abhorrence towards a technological imperative to maintain life at all costs. In Chapter II this problem is addressed in an attempt to separate arguments for and against euthanasia, by either act or omission, from proposals to limit, or abate, therapy. It is important to maintain this distinction, especially in the light of the growing momentum in favour of patient autonomy, where mechanisms are being considered for patient decision-making concerning therapy at the end-stages of life. Recognition of autonomous refusal of therapy, it is argued, need not be seen as a step towards euthanasia and must be separated from appeals to patient autonomy as a justification of euthanasia. The problem with linking autonomous refusal of therapy with euthanasia is considered towards the end of Chapter II, in a brief review of the Netherlands' euthanasia programme.

There are a number of themes which appear in almost every chapter of this book; they can be expressed in terms of a concern with the problem of euthanasia, the prospect of real autonomy and concern with some of the beliefs about the mechanisms which purport to communicate autonomous decisions. Many of the underlying assumptions concerning the market model of health-care will be questioned. Of particular concern is a view of autonomy which reflects the choices of some abstract consumer-patient and formal mechanisms for the expression of these choices, of which it might be said bear as little relevance to moral decision-making as the meaningless consumer questionnaires and charters, which proliferate in the service industries.

Chapter III examines advance directives and living wills. These mechanisms have evolved as a means of enabling patients to give advance indication of therapy options during the end stages of life. It is argued in Chapter III that whilst they are prone to misunderstanding and possible abuse, advance directives which specify a limit to life-prolonging therapy should be wholly separated from proposals for euthanasia. Charges of potential abuse can be met if patients and doctors share knowledge of alternative therapy options and societal prejudice against disability is both recognised and combatted. Nevertheless, it is maintained that public scepticism towards advance directives has some legitimacy, since they are for the most part unsatisfactory expressions of autonomy and are best limited to a minority of people with strong beliefs rather than promoted as a public ideal.

Chapters IV and V address ethical problems concerning the withholding of therapeutic intervention. Whilst Chapter IV examines the problems raised by proposals to withhold cardiopulmonary resuscitation, Chapter V focuses on the broader topic of medical futility and the related issue of physician autonomy. The moral status of withholding nutrition and hydration from patients in persistent vegetative states is considered in Chapter VI, and proposals to withhold expensive therapy are considered in Chapter VII. The final two chapters focus on the application of the principle of respect for autonomy, and it is argued that other moral demands should provide limits to autonomous refusal of therapy.

Of primary importance throughout this book is a recognition of a need to bridge the gap between respect for the principle of autonomy on the one hand and respect for the principle of beneficence on the other. Of course, when appeals to self-determination and best interests coincide there is no ethical problem. But the philosophical task of exposing hidden assumptions and potential conflicts can highlight actual and potential situations where a physician's values concerning what is best for the patient conflict with the latter's preference for certain therapy options. In some cases a patient may decline therapy which a doctor feels morally obliged to provide. More recently there have been cases where patients or their families have demanded therapy which their doctors regard as morally objectionable to provide. This conflict has been traditionally presented as a clash between patient autonomy and physician paternalism. For almost thirty years philosophers and bioethicists have, in general, supported arguments which place greater value on patient autonomy. Some of the mechanisms devised to promote patient autonomy have, however, created further ethical problems as well as risks of abuse and the potential curtailment of health-care for those who need it. In short, the autonomy movement has apparently run into difficulties. What is needed is some form of higher ethical synthesis of the principles of self-determination and recognition of the moral validity of the physician's perception of a patient's best interests. Throughout this book this synthesis is referred to as a principle of limited paternalism: it recognises that doctors and health-care professionals are moral agents whose professional expertise is necessarily permeated with moral values, and that these moral values must be taken seriously alongside respect for the dignity and autonomy of patients. Neither patient autonomy nor physician autonomy should be given exclusive priority in any moral conflict. In fact, the attempt to prioritise these principles is one of the weaknesses of the engineering or foundational model discussed in the early part of this chapter. Exponents of the engineering model assume that conflicts between patient self-determination and the physician's perception of beneficence can be settled within philosophical discourse. Instead, it will be argued throughout the following chapters that the interplay between patient and physician autonomy is context-dependant and that moral arguments in favour of either patient autonomy or the doctor's duty to act beneficently may achieve greater or less significance according to the context. What matters, then, is not the basic principles themselves but how our duties in relation to them are negotiated and interpreted.

II Therapy Abatement and Euthanasia

Introduction

Many arguments in favour of euthanasia rely on examples of life-prolonging therapy applied to unwilling patients in circumstances which suggest that a dignified death is being denied to those whose suffering is unnecessarily extended. In this respect requests for the withdrawal of certain life-prolonging procedures is presented as an inseparable issue from requests for euthanasia or 'mercy killing'. Similarly, a patient's expression of an autonomous decision regarding therapy options is frequently regarded as morally equivalent to an autonomous decision in favour of assisted suicide. With increasing public demand for greater control over therapy options at the end of life, is it possible to separate current interest in legal directives which specify options to forego various forms of life-sustaining therapy from the 'right to die' and 'right to kill' objectives frequently expressed by pro-euthanasia pressure groups? Is an enlightened attitude towards autonomous decisions regarding therapy abatement likely to encourage steps towards voluntary or non-voluntary euthanasia? One of the overriding concerns of this chapter is the belief that unless we achieve greater clarity and understanding about the issues raised by decisions to withhold or refuse life-prolonging therapy we cannot be in a position to fend off moves towards the decriminalisation of euthanasia and a passive tolerance of non-voluntary euthanasia.

Therapy Abatement

In November, 1991, *The Hastings Center Report* referred to an invitation to President George Bush to attend the funeral of a 'hard working and patriotic American'. The invitation included a request for the President to make a convenient date known, so the family could terminate the proposed decedent's life-support to accommodate the President's schedule. It was thought unlikely that the President would accept, but the example illustrates some of the confusion likely to occur in the context of proposals to give patients and/or their surrogates greater control over the dying process. There are however cases where the timing of death has been manipulated for non-medical reasons. In 1986 it came to light that the death of King George V was due to a drug overdose administered by his physician. His life was shortened by a few hours. One reason given was that the doctor thought that news of his death would be better reported in the *Times* than in the *Evening News*.

Fears of medical technology out of control are well-expressed in Robert F. Weir's (1990) appraisal of therapy options for the terminally ill. He speaks of the need to 'establish reasonable ethical limits to the technological prolongation of life lest we become unthinking and uncaring slaves to that technology'. (Weir, 1990:viii) Weir's arguments and case studies should be placed in the context of recent legislation in the USA on living wills, advance directives and legal directives on treatment abatement cases, including decisions to abate technological feeding and hydration. But these are also ethical issues of universal concern.

The legitimacy of government interest in sustaining life is beyond dispute, as it is fundamental to the criminal law. The question is whether or not it is compelling in the case of an individual's interest in rejecting life-prolonging therapy. Of particular importance to the question of distinguishing euthanasia from withdrawal of therapy is Weir's concept of 'treatment abatement', which means - in one crucial sense - 'decisions to withhold', or not to initiate a form of treatment, and also a 'reduction in degree or intensity' or 'a progressive diminishing of treatment'. (Weir, 1990:10) A further meaning is 'nullification' or 'termination', which encompasses 'decisions by autonomous, critically ill or terminally ill patients (or the surrogates of non-autonomous patients) to refuse all forms of life-sustaining treatment'. (*ibid*:10) Whilst this latter case is close to euthanasia, it nevertheless embraces those conditions where inevitable death is recognised - and hence the futility of life-prolonging therapy is apparent - whilst a moral imperative to provide comfort and care is uppermost. Withdrawal of some - but not all - forms of therapy need not be synonymous with euthanasia, especially when treating the terminally ill. There are limits to therapy abatement; refusing surgery may still leave the patient with the option of palliative care. However, the refusal of nursing care may require discharge from the hospital, which has an obligation to provide standards of hygiene, which include bathing and changing of clothes. The refusal of nursing care is not an option for the exercise of autonomy within the hospital.

Calls for therapy abatement raise serious moral arguments when they are made in contexts where the provision of 'life-sustaining therapy' is either contemplated or has been initiated. Life-sustaining therapy can be defined as any medical therapy administered to a patient in order to forestall the moment of death, whether or not the therapy is intended to treat any underlying cause of the life-threatening disease. Such forms of therapy might include, ventilators, dialysis and cardiopulmonary resuscitation. It must be stressed that the withdrawal or foregoing of forms of life-sustaining therapy is not equivalent to the withdrawal of *all* treatment.

The withdrawal or withholding of therapy which has proved to be useless in the face of inevitable death has always been an aspect of 'good medical practice' and should not be construed as 'mercy killing' - either by act or omission. Informed religious opinion recognises that it is good medical practice to allow death to occur at an appropriate time. The Roman Catholic Church issued a *Declaration On Euthanasia* (Sacred Congregation of the Doctrine of the Faith, 1980) which stated that 'The Church does not insist that a dying or seriously ill person should be kept alive by all possible means for as long as possible. The treatment should be proportionate to the therapeutic effect to be expected, and should not be disproportionately painful, intrusive, risky and costly in the circumstances.' A similar statement was issued by the Christian Medical Fellowship to the House of Lords Select Committee on Medical Ethics: (1994:15-16) 'we see no requirement to give all possible treatment to all possible patients in all possible situations because those treatments exist. It is precisely this sort of meddlesome medicine which does not recognise that the natural end is drawing near that has led to over-treatment of some patients.... a time may come when interventionist treatment need not be started or continued, and the patient should be allowed to die.'

It is sometimes misleading to speak of 'letting die' by withdrawing certain forms of therapy from the terminally ill. In some cases there is nothing else a doctor can do. The expression 'I let him die' has a meaning only if there is a possible chance of maintaining life. When facing inevitable death the choice is not between life and death, but how the patient shall die. For this reason outmoded discussions about the relative moral weight that should be attached to either actions which shorten life and omissions which shorten life, or discussions concerning the distinction between extraordinary and non-extraordinary therapy, are of little relevance to the consideration of therapy options for terminal patients. It should be stressed that 'therapy abatement' is not synonymous with 'termination of all therapy'. Properly understood, it captures that aspect of sound medical practice which recognises that there are times when the dying process should be rendered more comfortable. It is widely held that there is no ethical imperative to subject a patient to repeated attempts at resuscitation, a futile regime of intravenous alimentation, dialysis, drug-dependent maintenance of the blood pressure 'prophylactic' antibiotics, and control of the heartbeat by electrical means in order to maintain survival for a couple of days, or even a week, and that it is more important to concentrate on physical comfort where therapy might involve more emphasis on oral hygiene, and care of skin in a family environment outside the ICU. Thus to avoid confusion between therapy abatement and euthanasia (passive or active) it is important to place emphasis on a distinction between a doctor's respective duties, between 'treating for living' and 'treating for dying'. (Kennedy, 1988)

There are times, in the course of treating terminally ill patients (or anencephalic infants with no hope of any future), when treatment for dying is the only morally appropriate course, and where the infliction of life-prolonging therapy *is* morally unjustifiable. This point is expressed by Robert Twycross and Sylvia Lack in their study of therapy options for patients suffering from advanced cancer.

> Nasogastric tubes, intravenous infusions, antibiotics, cardiac resuscitation and artificial respiration are all primarily supportive measures for use in acute or acute-on-chronic illness to assist a patient through the initial period towards recovery of health. To use such measures in patients who are close to death and have no expectancy of a return to health is generally inappropriate, and therefore bad medicine. (Twycross and Lack, 1986:7)

Under appropriate conditions it is good medical practice to treat severely brain-damaged infants (for example, anencephalics) as dying patients, rather than engage in hopeless and futile attempts to prolong their lives. Such a course should not be confused with proposals for the 'mercy killing' of newborns, which was advocated by Singer and Kuhse (1985). There is, however, an urgent need for open discussion and guidelines regarding the categories of severely disabled newborns for whom treatment for dying should supersede attempts at life-prolongation. It is well established in both law and ethics that efforts should not be made to prolong life in any condition. This was apparent in the case of *Baby J*, (1990) where the House of Lords rejected an absolute sanctity of life standpoint.

On the 28 May, 1990, an infant boy, known as Baby J, was born in England. He had a limited life expectancy. He was 13 weeks premature, weighing two and a half pounds, was brain-damaged, paralysed, probably blind and deaf, incapable of spontaneous breathing such that life could only be maintained with the aid of a ventilator for the first month of his life. But after three unsuccessful attempts to wean him from the ventilator he eventually became capable of spontaneous respiration. Concern was expressed over the possibility that with future chest infections, reventilation would even worsen his quality of life. Baby J was made a ward of court and in October 1990 the Court of Appeal ruled that further attempts at life- prolongation were not in his best interests. The Law Lords upheld the view that further mechanical ventilation should not be provided in the event of Baby J stopping breathing as it would likely cause greater distress, adding to an already appalling catalogue of disabilities. (*Baby J*, 1990) Lord Justice Taylor said that the case had created a 'hideous dilemma', but he emphasised that the courts could never sanction steps to terminate a life. (Reported in *The Independent*, 20 October, 1990:6). An editorial in *The Sunday Correspondent*, 21 October, 1990:18) saw that judgement as an endorsement of 'current medical practice'. On the other hand, pro-life organizations expressed fears that the courts were actually endorsing euthanasia and offers were made to provide life-prolonging therapy for Baby J. The case showed a clear need for an informed debate on this issue which raised moral issues which went beyond disputes over medical knowledge, such as the value society places on the quality of life.

Another case, that of *Baby C* (1989), indicated that both legal and medical opinion is concerned primarily with duties to provide appropriate medical treatment rather than the technological prolongation of life. Baby C was born prematurely on 23 December, 1988 and was suffering from a severe form of hydrocephalus which had seriously impaired her brain structure. An operation was performed to remove the pressure on her brain. This operation is often done with hydrocephalus with good results. But in this case the damage to her brain was already irreparable. At best the operation prevented enlargement of her head, thus rendering her some relief. Due to uncertainty over future treatment or the withholding of life-prolonging treatment, Baby C was made a ward of court. The question facing the courts concerned what future treatment she should receive if she succumbed to future life-threatening illnesses over and above her disabilities. For example, should she be given antibiotics if she succumbed to a respiratory disease that would otherwise cause her death? The court recognised that she had received the best treatment appropriate to her condition that the country could offer. When the issue came before the Law Lords two alternatives were considered: should she receive future treatment, as one social worker testified, 'appropriate to a non-handicapped child', or as the legal department of the local authority held, should she 'receive such treatment as is appropriate to her condition'? Lord Donaldson, Master of the Rolls, took the latter view. The Lords sought advice from a senior paediatrician who said, after an examination of Baby C, that her disability was even worse than had previously been described and that there was no hope for any improvement in her condition. Acting on the expert's advice the Lords took the view that 'the goal should be to ease the suffering of Baby C rather than to achieve a short prolongation of her life'. This view, of course, depended on the judgement that Baby C was actually dying, and therapy abatement was justified on the grounds that undue prolongation was not in her best interests. Thus by regarding her as dying, not just disabled, the question was *how* she should die, not whether she should be allowed to die by either act or omission. This decision, which effectively limited certain forms of intervention to prolong her life, left open questions concerning incompetent patients who are disabled but not dying.

There are few precedents in English law concerning therapy abatement decisions for competent adults. However, several recent cases have received attention and indicate the direction in which legal and ethical opinion appears to be moving. The first case, *Re T*, (1992) involved a 20 year old woman, Miss T, who was admitted to hospital following a road traffic accident on 4 July, 1992. She was 34 weeks pregnant. On 5 July, when she was in considerable pain, and suffering contractions in the early stages of labour, a decision was taken that the delivery should be by caesarian section. Although Miss T was not at the time a Jehovah's Witness she had been brought up by her mother who was a fervent member of that faith. Following a visit from her mother Miss T refused consent to a blood transfusion. When her condition deteriorated she was sent to intensive care. With further signs of deterioration the hospital authorities decided that it would be in her best interests to receive a transfusion, which was carried out on 8 July. When the case came before the Law Lords, Lord Donaldson, Master of the

Rolls, noted that whilst 'she was undoubtedly under the influence of her mother, she was capable of reaching and did reach a decision as to her own treatment'. Lord Donaldson added:

> An adult patient who...suffers from no mental incapacity has an absolute right to choose whether to consent to medical treatment, to refuse it or to choose one rather than another of the treatments being offered....This right of choice is not limited to decisions which others might regard as sensible. It exists notwithstanding that the reasons for making the choice are rational, irrational, unknown or even non-existent.

Lord Donaldson then set out conditions which would ensure that therapy refusal was legally binding. These conditions require that the patient had full mental capacity at the time the decision was made, was under no undue influence, and that the patient understood the consequences of refusing therapy.

A second case, *Re C*, (1993) which was widely discussed in the press, (*The Guardian*, 15 October, 1993) involved a chronic paranoid schizophrenic male patient suffering from delusions of grandeur at Broadmoor Hospital who had a gangrenous leg which his doctors had proposed to amputate from below the knee. The patient, Mr. C., refused to consent to the operation. The hospital trust refused to undertake not to operate were he to become incompetent in the future. However, a High Court ruling held that Mr. C. was competent to make a decision concerning the proposed treatment, and that his refusal of amputation complied with Lord Donaldson's test, and that Mr. C's. decision should be binding even if he should become incompetent. An injunction was granted to prevent treatment.

In the case of *Airedale NHS Trust v Bland*, involving a request for the discontinuation of life-prolonging therapy for a young man in a persistent vegetative state, Lord Goff indicated that subject to certain conditions an anticipatory refusal of treatment should be binding: 'it has never been held,' said Lord Goff, 'that a patient of sound mind may, if properly informed, require that life support should be discontinued... the same principle applies where the patient's refusal to give his consent has been expressed at an earlier date, before he became unconscious or otherwise incapable of communicating it'.

These cases indicate a shift in legal thinking in favour of both immediate and prior refusal of treatment, a view recently echoed in the Law Commission's evidence to the House of Lords Select Committee on Medial Ethics (1994:39) which regarded advance directives to forego certain therapeutic procedures as 'recognised at common law, which does not permit treatment to be provided which the patient has previously refused.' The Select Committee accepted this position and expressed an opinion which endorsed the right of a competent patient to refuse *any* medical treatment for whatever reason. However, the Select Committee insisted that this is 'far removed from the right to request assistance in dying' (*ibid*:48) and saw the prohibition of intentional killing as the cornerstone of law and of social relationships. Nevertheless, the Select Committee did express misgivings over proposals to enable proxies or surrogates to make decisions on behalf of incompetent patients.

The context in which therapy is provided often determines the ethical imperatives regarding therapy options. In hospices and nursing homes for the elderly the moral imperative to prolong life is not uppermost - as it may be in an ICU or accident unit. Yet even here treatment abatement, in the sense of 'not initiating' or 'diminishing' therapy, does not amount to euthanasia. The central philosophy of the hospice movement is the need to maximise the quality, not necessarily the quantity, of remaining life, and if life-prolongation involves the infliction of suffering it is not regarded as an ultimate good to be sought at all costs. The point of hospice care is not the addition of more days but the prolongation of an ability to make each day count for something. A similar imperative is relevant for nursing homes for the elderly where 'Do not resuscitate' orders and 'Do not hospitalise' orders may be morally acceptable. Given the average age of 82 years in nursing homes for the elderly, removal to a hospital may be confusing, and unsettling, so ending one's days in comfort may have greater value than life-prolongation. Thus in the context of geriatric care 'appropriate medical practice does not always mean employing all the guns of medical technology'. (A physician cited by Weir, 1990:50)

It has been argued here that various forms of therapy abatement, even when life-threatening, are compatible with principles of good medical practice and respect for the individual. When properly addressed decisions regarding therapy abatement should replace arguments about euthanasia, as the essential moral argument is over which form of therapy is ethically appropriate, not whether continued life is ethically appropriate. But although euthanasia is incompatible with the principles of good medical practice, the infliction of life-prolonging therapy which merely increases suffering is equally objectionable. Whilst the strongest case in favour of euthanasia may be the alleviation of suffering, opponents of euthanasia should not find it necessary to argue in favour of the infliction of suffering in order to maintain life at all costs. It is sometimes argued that suffering, which may be of no benefit to the patient, has a value in that it benefits others. Thus John J. O'Connor (1989) [Cardinal] appeals to the value of suffering:

> A frightening number of people are being condemned to death by the courts, at the request of loved ones or 'proxies', or by their own personal requests. The reason: They are suffering 'needlessly'; their lives are 'useless'; they are terminally ill or comatose, or 'have nothing to live for'. What an enormous difference it could make to such patients or to those acting on their behalf, if they understood the power of suffering.....those suffering unto death merit our thanking them for their testimony to life - and for helping us save our souls.

This argument is merely the mirror image of euthanasia for the unwanted. The sufferer is treated as a means for someone else's objectives, even if, in this case the objective is the moral elevation of others. Undoubtedly awareness of suffering helps us understand the suffering of others and it can be morally elevating to witness suffering borne with courage. But this kind of suffering cannot be inflicted upon those who do not want to accept it, and whatever value it may have it should not override a free and autonomous decision not to be a moral hero. Suffering is a virtue, but it can be so only if accepted freely with patience and resignation.

Killing and Letting Die

The line between therapy abatement and euthanasia has often been blurred by discussions over the relationship between actions which bring about death (killing) and inactions which lead to death (letting die). Thus many proponents of euthanasia describe the distinction between active and passive euthanasia, killing and letting die, as morally irrelevant, and then go on to equate the withdrawal or withholding of life-sustaining therapy as morally similar to active euthanasia. An abstract appeal to consequences, unrelated to the context in which therapy is either applied, withheld, or withdrawn, might very well suggest that these distinctions are merely semantical. But a closer look at the *context* in which therapy decisions are made suggests that many of the arguments and examples cited which are designed to shift attention to the consequences of an act or omission have little moral significance and frequently represent an artificial intrusion of a simplistic philosophical dogma into medical ethics.

The following example should indicate why most health-care professionals make a distinction between killing and withholding life-prolonging therapy. A patient with respiratory failure may or may not be put on a ventilator. The appropriateness of the action would depend on whether the therapy was deemed futile, or whether the patient had expressly requested not to receive ventilation. In short, the outcome would be assessed according to the background and related circumstances. But a doctor who uses a pillow to suffocate a patient is clearly guilty of homicide whatever the context.

There has been, in recent years, both an ethical and legal shift in favour of medical aid-in-dying, which is a form of euthanasia. This has been shown in an increasing reluctance to prosecute and convict a growing number of health-care professionals who have actively brought about their patient's deaths. In several cases the line between active termination of life and the withholding of therapy has been blurred. A recent Canadian Supreme Court action sparked off a considerable debate on the morality of physician-assisted suicide. The issue involved the death of Ms. Sue Rodriguez in February, 1994, who suffered from amyotrophic lateral sclerosis (ALS) and whose death, it was alleged, involved the help of a doctor. Ms. Rodriguez had previously had her plea for physician-assisted suicide refused by a 5 to 4 ruling which attracted media attention. A Canadian opinion poll, asking whether doctor-assisted suicide should be legally permitted, found 74% in favour, 21% against and 5% unsure. (Spooner, 1994:2) Another much publicised example involves Dr. Jack Kevorkian, a retired USA pathologist, who has used a 'suicide machine' on several patients. This machine is constructed so as to allow the patient to perform the final act. He continued to use his machine despite an injunction issued by a Michigan court and the revocation of his medical licence. Several years ago an anonymous author published in the *Journal of the American Medical Association*, a piece entitled 'Its Over Debbie'. The author claimed to be a physician who had injected morphine sulphate sedative to cause the death of a patient. Despite a search for the author no prosecution followed. According to Lawrence O. Gostin (1993) these examples indicate of a shift in moral attitudes towards physician-assisted suicide.

Nevertheless, these examples would be seen as instances of causing rather than allowing death. The moral weight, so it would seem, apparently falling upon the notions of intentionality and causality. This is precisely the view advanced by Edmund D. Pellegrino (1993) who argues that in active euthanasia the doctor intentionally causes the patient's death, whereas in foregoing treatment, the disease causes the patient's death. But Howard Brody (1993) argues that the appeal to intention or causality does not adequately maintain the moral distinction between acting and omitting. Brody cites several compelling examples, including medical negligence where the doctor's failure to act leads to a patient's death despite no evidence that death was intended or actively caused. In this case it would be the disease which killed the patient, but were the doctor put on trial for negligence, an appeal on this ground would not succeed. The negligent doctor can be culpable without intending to kill or cause death, as he has an obligation to treat where appropriate.

Nevertheless, there are powerful reasons for maintaining a distinction between the withholding of certain forms of life-prolonging treatment and causing death. It is important to retain an awareness that discussions about what kind of therapy can be withheld or provided belong to a different moral category than arguments about allowing or causing death. In fact a consideration of a situation where there was no recognisable difference between withholding therapy and killing reveals the inherent weakness of the opposing position. The implications of rejecting the moral distinction between therapy abatement and the administration of a lethal injection can be seen if we take the argument literally. It would require a situation where medical treatment was so successful that death from any disease, or from natural causes, has been eliminated, and doctors, like Gods, could themselves decide whether someone should live or die. In such a situation the only cause of death would be the termination of treatment or the administration of poison. It would also require a situation such that whenever a doctor decided that a treatment was futile the next obvious step is to administer a lethal dose, as a quick direct killing is the only logical course. Such a position, if it were the case, would rest on the assumption that doctors had tremendous powers and knowledge, including the ability to postpone the death of their patients for an unlimited period.

The mistake in arguments which deny any difference between

therapy abatement and direct killing is found in their excessive concern with the consequences of an action and a tendency to overlook, not only the intentions behind it but the context in which it was considered. As Daniel Callaghan (1992:53) points out, it also involves a confusion between causality and culpability, a misunderstanding of the way our society has 'overlaid natural causes with moral rules and interpretations'. The notion of 'causality' applies to the direct cause of death, whereas 'culpability' refers to the attribution of moral responsibility to actions. Thus, for example, causality and culpability are confused when the actions of a doctor in ceasing life-sustaining therapy is construed as causing death. When a doctor withholds or withdraws therapy and the patient dies, it is the *disease* which *causes* death, the culpability of the doctor remains a matter of contingency. The doctor would be culpable, for example, if a patient had a good chance of survival which was forestalled because the therapy was deliberately withheld or withdrawn or in the examples cited by Brody (1993) where criminal negligence was an issue.

The language of killing/letting die or acts/omissions fails to capture the moral problems. Discovering and establishing differences between active and passive causal roles does not adequately address the moral requirement to determine when one set of duties should replace another set of duties. Moreover, when determining culpability one may discover that the conceptual distinction between acts and omissions does not carry the moral weight that is placed upon it. It cannot replace the need to examine each case on its merit. A doctor would be culpable if she administered a lethal combination of drugs and might also be culpable if she failed to intervene in circumstances where a death could have been prevented. But the doctor would not be culpable if the therapy was withheld on the grounds that it was futile or likely to cause harm to the patient. No doctor can be said to be culpable if she gives up in the recognition of defeat. Culpability, then, is bound up with the moral judgements which are appropriately called for when assessing the reasons for either action or inaction. Omitted actions do not always have the same moral status as actions bound up with intentional killing or professional negligence. Letting someone die may involve carelessness and callousness, but it is not homicide, although there may be degrees of culpability according to the agents' professional responsibilities. Nevertheless, if the intention is to kill, then any act or omission designed to fulfil this objective will be morally identical. Leaving the issue of negligence aside there is an important difference between a moral responsibility for an action and a causal responsibility for it. To be morally responsible for an action one must intend the consequences for which it is causally responsible. It should be stressed in this context that the location of intentionality is not as difficult as it is often held to be: even a dog knows the difference between an intentional kick and being carelessly tripped over.

Many investigations have concluded that it is difficult to maintain a clear-cut conceptual difference between action and inaction and their consequences. The actress who gives a third rate performance may wreck the play, just as she would if she had not turned up at the theatre. There may be little difference in educational results between a method of directed teaching and leaving the student to find out for himself. It is the same with regard to the provision of therapy; the difference between causing and allowing something to happen, or more specifically, killing and letting die is equally hard to maintain. What ought to be concluded from examinations of the distinction between acts and omissions is not that acts are *morally* equivalent to omissions, but that the distinctions do not carry the moral weight that is placed upon them, and it should also be stressed in this context that arguments designed to collapse these distinctions, such that action is deemed to be morally equivalent to inaction, also fail to establish the moral guidelines that are frequently held to be derived from them. For example, James Rachels (1986) proposes a defence of euthanasia which rests on the collapse of the acts-omissions distinction. He argues that in many circumstances passive non-intervention may lead to greater wrong than actively killing. One of his examples concerns a terminally ill patient where therapy would be worse than actively killing him, as 'it will take him longer to die, and so he will suffer *more* than if we administer the lethal injection.' (*Ibid*:108-9) Yet all this argument really shows is that the acts and omissions distinction does not provide a basis for moral judgement about rightful and wrongful killing; it does not provide a justification for euthanasia or a condemnation of it. This is because moral judgements about rightful and wrongful killing have priority over conceptual distinctions between activity and inactivity. Distinctions about rightful and wrongful killing do not rest upon conceptual distinctions between passivity and activity but on our understanding of what circumstances prohibit or permit killing. Thus, for example, we recognize that killing in self-defence is morally permissible, either by actively overpowering assailants or by remaining passive when they fall off the rooftop/or sink in the swamp/or set fire to themselves in the course of their murderous attempts. The issue here is not how the assailant dies, but whether his death is permissible. The distinction between rightful and wrongful killing will have to be established independently of distinctions between action and inaction.

We have argued that the extent of culpability in medical practice is bound up with the manner in which moral responsibility is attributed to either actions or inactions. This in turn is to be understood with reference to the actual duties which are deemed appropriate in certain circumstances in particular stages during the course of a patient's illness. In this respect a duty to combine respect for patient autonomy with a beneficial imperative may involve a daily re-assessment of what kind of therapy should be withheld or provided, and this could very well involve numerous moral dilemmas which are not simply reducible to a killing-letting die, active-passive euthanasia distinction.

A borderline example is the over-prescribing of potentially lethal drugs to terminally ill patients. According to Robert A. Sedler (1993) the whole business of decriminalising euthanasia, securing amendments to statutes which permit physician-assisted 'aids-in-dying' by means of lethal injection, the controversy over assisted suicide and recourse to Dr. Kevorkian's suicide machine, could be circumvented if a terminally ill patient is prescribed a sufficient amount of pain-killing drugs in such quantities as to empower her to hasten an inevitable death. The act would be carried out by the patient at her own time not requiring a visit from the doctor or anyone with an interest in participating in another's suicide. In such cases, argues Sedler, the doctor would not have acted in order to kill, would not have administered a lethal dose, but would have prescribed pain-killing drugs which the patient may decide to take as directed by the doctor or in sufficient quantities to accelerate an inevitable death.

It is likely that this kind of proposal raises as many problems as it apparently solves. Where, for example, does one draw the line between a genuinely compassionate desire to relieve suffering and empower the patient with some final control over her destiny and an act of moral blackmail which a distressed patient perceives as a strong hint that she has become a nuisance and must 'do the honourable thing'? Quite clearly no blue-prints can be supplied for such situations, and the moral status of the doctor's decision would be relative to the nature of the relationship between doctor and patient. It is worth noting a remark made by a spokesperson for the British Geriatrics Society in evidence to the House of Lords Select Committee on Medical Ethics (1994:26) 'although elderly severely ill patients may sometimes ask to be allowed to die, they very seldom request active procedures to ensure that they do.'

But what is clear in such examples is the limited nature of moral discourse which rests on an appeal to the consequences of either acts and omissions. Ian Kennedy (1988:324) quite rightly rejects this approach and emphasises that decisions should be taken in the light of perceived duties. A doctor, he argues, has a duty to preserve life and a duty to care for dying patients and make them comfortable. A point may come in the course of a patient's illness when one duty supersedes another: when the duty to retain physical functions increases the physical discomfort of the dying patient it is time to conform with the duty to provide comfort and care. Thus antibiotics for pneumonia would not be ethically indicated, argues Kennedy, if the patient were to survive for a further period of discomfort, pain and disintegration. The same argument applies to the withholding or withdrawal of ventilatory support, an issue which has been unnecessarily complicated by misleading and emotive references to 'switching off' and 'pulling the plug'. If a patient requires a ventilator then a doctor has an obligation to ventilate, but if ventilation is of no benefit and would prolong a life of discomfort, then the doctor has no duty to ventilate, and the death of the patient would not be the result of either withholding or withdrawing ventilatory support, but of the disease process which - despite all efforts - the doctor is unable to cure.

In many cases confusion has reigned because the moral questions have not been put forward correctly. Too often the question has been formulated in terms of whether or not the patient should be allowed to die, or whether or not a life should be prolonged. This form of question moves the issue very close to deliberations on physician-assisted suicide. But the important moral and medical questions are bound up with the doctor's duties: does the doctor have a duty to continue the life of a patient by means of this or that therapy or is it in the best interests of the patient and in accord with professional standards of health-care, that a life should not be continued by means of a certain form of therapy? Moral discourse about duties may embrace a wide range of therapeutic options for a seriously ill or terminally ill patient and is certainly not reducible to simplistic slogans about killing and letting die.

The key moral and legal questions must be determined by an understanding of the doctor's duty to a patient. In his summary to the jury in *R v Bodkin Adams*, ([1957] Crim. L.R. 365) Devlin J. said:

> If the first purpose of medicine, the restoration of health, can no longer be achieved there is still very much for a doctor to do, and he is entitled to do all that is proper and

necessary to relieve pain and suffering, even if the measures he takes may incidentally shorten life.

This was by no means an advocacy for euthanasia or physician-assisted suicide, but a statement which recognised that some attempts at life-prolongation may be futile, and that once this is established then the doctor must consider other duties bound up with the relief of suffering and distress. Once this is established then no charge of euthanasia, by either act or omission, could be made. This acknowledgement of the doctor's duties is built into the special role society bestows upon doctors in their dispensation of drugs and therapeutic interventions.

Medical duties are guided by references to a patient's best interests. There is no moral difference between failing to start and stopping a course of therapy already started, as long as both decisions are taken with reference to the patient's best interests. A set of circumstances which justifies not starting would justify stopping a course of therapy. If this point is accepted then the employment of a therapy on a trial basis need not be restricted by potential reluctance to stop it if it becomes obviously futile at a later stage. In evidence submitted to the House of Lords Select Committee on Medical Ethics (1994:16) the BMA endorsed this point: 'for all practical purposes it was important that doctors should feel able to withdraw treatment which was not producing benefits for the patient. They could thus in an emergency situation initiate all potentially beneficial interventions, confident that the regime could be reviewed later.' Likewise, the British Geriatric Society insisted how 'it is very important that doctors should not be constrained in offering possibly beneficial treatment by the thought that they would not have the right to discontinue if it were not benefiting the patient.' (*ibid*:16). For example, in an emergency situation one may employ ventilatory support without adequate time to assess its potential futility. An awareness that it is not a moral failure to withdraw futile therapy would therefore overcome any resistance to 'having a go' with potentially salvageable patients. Nevertheless, there is a feeling, often expressed, that once started discontinuation of therapy carries a burden of guilt; it may be preferable - except in emergencies - to consider the situation and decide not to initiate therapy. When deciding whether or not to initiate or withhold a form of therapy the doctor should be guided by her prognostic skills but, from the doctor's standpoint, the moral justification of any chosen course lies in the duty to the patient's best interests. As we have seen, however, a duty to protect a patient's best interests is modified with reference to the importance society attaches to patient autonomy and consent to treatment.

The Netherlands: A Slippery Slope?

The practice of euthanasia in the Netherlands has been subjected to rigorous examination. Whilst many proponents of euthanasia see this as an enlightened step, there are others who have expressed serious misgivings. This section will examine some of the issues raised in the debate over euthanasia in the Netherlands.

In February, 1993, the Dutch Parliament gave formal approval to the practice of euthanasia, provided that evidence is provided of the patient's 'persistent' request. In the Netherlands there are no procedures for euthanasia by means of advance directives or by proxy. Only current requests are legally permitted.

The definition of euthanasia in law and medicine in the Netherlands is 'the active termination of a patient's life at his or her request, by a physician'. The underpinning ethical principle appears to be based on respect for the free informed decisions made by a rational individual. Euthanasia is strictly speaking, illegal, but legally tolerated. Dutch law has a distinctive doctrine concerning certain practices that are statutorily illegal but tolerated (*gedogen*) by the public prosecutor and the courts. This allows practices to evolve by toleration before they are made legal. Then, when a consensus emerges, a law can be passed to regulate the practice as it has evolved. This is markedly different to the UK and USA where there is a tendency to address a social issue initially with a law which may then be amended in the light of public reaction. Thus, in the case of tolerated euthanasia, doctors who adhere to three conditions, recognised by the courts and sanctioned by the state, will not be prosecuted. These are: 1] the patient's request must be voluntary, persistent and conscious; 2] the patient must exhibit unbearable suffering, which cannot be relieved by any other means; 3] the attending physician must consult with a colleague regarding the genuineness of 1 and 2, and the appropriateness of euthanasia.

It is believed by the Dutch medical and legal authorities - although there are many dissenting voices (Fenigsen, 1989) - that these safeguards provide a sufficient defence against abuse, preventing further steps in the direction of non-voluntary euthanasia. However, two questions arise: the first question is whether or not the guidelines can effectively hold the euthanasia programme to the killing of those who rationally desire to be killed, and the second question is whether it is desired that these guidelines should function as an effective brake or merely function as a device to meet objections whilst gradually introducing more widespread forms of euthanasia. It would seem, from recent investigations into the practice of euthanasia in the Netherlands, that the guidelines are not effective in preventing non-voluntary euthanasia and that a more widespread commitment to euthanasia appears to be lurking in the background. (Keown, 1992)

Not all cases have involved repeated requests from the patients. On 5 July, 1994 John Carvel reported in *The Guardian* that a four-day-old Dutch baby suffering from hydrocephalus and an exposed spinal chord was given a lethal injection by her doctor following consultations with several paediatricians and neurologists. On a strict interpretation of Dutch law this would have been illegal, as the guidelines do not specify whether euthanasia is permitted for severely deformed infants who are incapable of requesting it. There is, as *The Guardian* report indicated, a reluctance to impose sentences on Dutch doctors found guilty of violating the euthanasia guidelines.

With tacit approval of the state and the medical authorities the euthanasia programme has already overstepped its own criteria. A survey conducted by the Remmelink Committee, so named after Professor J. Remmelink, the Attorney General of the Dutch Supreme Court, who chaired the Committee in 1990-91, revealed that whilst the majority of cases examined conformed to the rules, in a significant number of cases the recommended criteria have not been enforced, and that non-voluntary euthanasia is practised with Government and societal approval. According to the Remmelink Committee (1991) in about 1000 cases of euthanasia in 1990 doctors intentionally accelerated death without a specific request from the patient. In 600 of these cases there was patient involvement, but for various reasons it had not reached the point of an explicit request.

Strictly speaking these 1000 cases violated Dutch law, which requires 'explicit request', although it is unlikely that a court would convict. (Van Delden Loes and Van der Maas, 1993:25) John Keown, who has been investigating euthanasia in the Netherlands, draws attention to other statistics and points out that in 'almost 5,000 of the 8,100 cases in which they intended to kill by administering opiates, the patient had not requested the hastening of death'. In short, he says, 'doctors stated that in 1990 they sought to accelerate death in some 20,000 cases, in almost three-quarters of which there had been no request by the patient'. (Keown, 1992:42) Giving evidence to the House of Lords Select Committee on Medical Ethics (1994:29) Keown criticised the Dutch criteria for euthanasia for its imprecision: for example, the requirement that 'request for euthanasia must come only from the patient and must be entirely free and voluntary' is not adequately defined. There is nothing to prevent a proposal for euthanasia being initially suggested by the doctor. Keown also said that the requirement that the request 'must be well considered, durable and persistent' is equally unspecific, and that in 13% of cases the interval between the first request and euthanasia is no more than a day. A further problem lies in the monitoring of euthanasia; as the facts of the case are reported by the doctors who perform the act they are unlikely to report cases which could lead to prosecution.

The Remmelink Report likewise revealed that at least one third of the 5000 or so patients who received a lethal dosage in 1991 did not give their unequivocal consent, and 400 never even raised the issue with their doctors, who admitted that their intention was to shorten lives, not alleviate pain. (Nowak, 1992) The House of Lords Select Committee on Medical Ethics (1994:67) noted the absence of palliative care in Dutch medical undergraduate training, and stated that the Netherlands were inferior to the UK's record in palliative care, drawing attention to a 1988 survey which revealed over 50% of patients with terminal cancer had their pain inadequately relieved, and 56% of Dutch doctors had inadequate knowledge of pain relief techniques. The Remmelink Report and various critics of the Netherlands' euthanasia programme, reveal that euthanasia, in this instance, has proved impossible to regulate. This raises questions whether there is sufficient will to regulate it anyhow, given a social background in which accelerated death is profitable, and there is pressure to eliminate certain categories of unwanted people. According to the Dutch Physician's League there are perceptions that a drive to save money on care of the elderly, demented and comatose, patients has played a role in the encouragement of euthanasia, and that whilst not explicit the desire to save resources was a major factor. (House of Lords Select Committee on Medical Ethics, 1994:66)

What appears to have happened in the Netherlands is that a programme which started on the basis of an appeal to individual autonomy, the right to a 'dignified death', whereby an individual could freely choose to surrender life when his or her condition became intolerable, has in practice capitulated to the authority of the medical profession, who, according to the Remmelink Committee, saw nothing troublesome in 1000 reported cases of non-voluntary euthanasia, which was justified on the grounds that the patient's doctors had decided for them that their suffering had become 'unbearable' and that their life must be considered 'given up', according to medical standards.

Commenting on the Netherlands' euthanasia programme, Henk A.M.J. ten Have and Jos V.M. Welie (1992:38) locate the origins of the dialectical reversal from patient autonomy to medical authority in recent history.

> In the 1970's the 'euthanasia movement' in the Netherlands began as a protest against the power of contemporary medicine to alienate individual's autonomy and control over his or her own life. It seems that social acceptance of euthanasia is resulting in physicians acquiring even more power over the life and death of their patients. As the Remmelink Report shows, in most cases of ending human life, it is the physician who decides that it is appropriate to hasten death.

This move from the primacy of patient autonomy to the surrender of autonomy to the medical profession is in part consequential upon the application of an abstract and simplistic concept of individual freedom which presupposes that decisions are meaningful independent of societal pressures and cultural beliefs.

It might be argued that evidence of abuse calls for greater education about euthanasia and stricter control over the criteria. This is hardly relevant in the Netherlands where intense education on this issue has been provided since the early 1970s, and the mechanisms for regulation are either ambiguous or not applied. In a special supplement to the *Hastings Center Report*, (March 1992) which focused upon euthanasia in the Netherlands, several critics hinted gravely of a hidden agenda, where doctors freely act on the belief that some people are better off dead.

Margaret Pabst Battin (1994) has written informatively about the Netherlands euthanasia programme which she considers as a model for legalised euthanasia in the USA. Whilst she recognises that abuses have taken place she nevertheless sees a beneficial side to the programme and compares the way euthanasia operates within Dutch society with the institution of marriage. Marriage is a voluntary institution of which society approves. It can be an arena of abuse and forced marriages are possible by means of blackmail or fear of violence. But we still support and cherish the institution of marriage whilst seeking to minimise abuse. So, she says, the same can be said of euthanasia in the Netherlands. The analogy has one fundamental limitation: abuse of the voluntary principle in marriage can always be rectified by annulment and divorce giving the victims a possibility of building a new life; with euthanasia there is no remedy and no life to rebuild.

Opponents of Dutch medical practice might argue that the Netherlands have begun a slippery slope which started with a justification of euthanasia strictly on the explicit request of a patient and then developed into a justification of non-requested deaths. It is, however, hard to establish a slippery slope in this instance as there is no hard data on the starting point. Such data could be provided if a survey of accelerated deaths had been conducted ten years ago. Nevertheless, a process appears to be under way whereby the justification of euthanasia was extended from an appeal to patient autonomy to an appeal to the doctor's moral beliefs. It might be noted that in the Netherlands, despite the alleged importance attributed to patient autonomy, it is often trumped by medical wisdom; two thirds of euthanasia requests are rejected by doctors (Deldon Loes, 1993). This would suggest that a criterion other than autonomy is being used.

Battin points out that the euthanasia programme in the Netherlands has emerged against a background of greater equality of access to healthcare than is available in the US in a society that is more tolerant of its composite social groups. There is less likelihood of abuse, she maintains, than in the US. Nevertheless, two lessons can be learnt from the Netherlands' experiment. First, in a climate in which there is profit in the elimination of unwanted people, and a significant proportion of influential people (particularly doctors) are committed to a programme of killing, then further steps down a slippery slope towards the killing of those who do not want to die is highly probable. (Lamb, 1988) Second, the Netherlands' experiment reveals how easy a society's commitment to individual autonomy can be surrendered once judgements like 'futility', 'unbearable', 'medically inappropriate', and that 'life has been ... given up' are regarded as purely clinical matters unrelated to moral discourse.

III Advance Directives and Living Wills

Introduction

The question addressed by proponents of living wills is the right to direct treatment during the end stages of one's life, especially when a stage is reached where one is no longer competent to make a rational decision. The media as well as the writings of many bioethicists have reported widespread fear of painful death in institutional isolation in circumstances where the disease process has severely limited the ability to make decisions concerning treatment options. A living will is a document upon which individuals can indicate in advance a preference not to be given various forms of therapy to prolong life. Living wills can also give directions for refusing specific forms of therapy, including blood transfusions, CPR, chemotherapy, renal dialysis, various intubations, ventilators, and nutrition and hydration. Many caring and compassionate institutions and individuals have supported them as a means of providing a patient with some means of control over his or her death, and extend personal autonomy into areas where the capacity to act autonomously is lost. Yet whilst the living will conveys a written expression of a person's desires it is difficult to imagine and comprehensively list all possible medical contingencies. Thus living wills are of limited value. Their precise interpretation may require further discussion with a doctor at a time when treatment decisions are to be taken. Hence in some American states durable powers of attorney statutes have emerged, whereby one can appoint an agent to act for oneself at any time after loss of the capacity for self-determination. In this respect the health-care power of attorney is a device to enable the patient to tell the doctor who the surrogate or proxy should be. Their legal force is stronger than living wills and in some states in the US the appointed agent's authority may overrule objections from family members. Taken together, 'living wills' or 'health-care powers of attorney' are known as 'advance directives.' Legal opinion in the UK, where laws are being considered to give further recognition to advance directives, is slightly different to the US. In England the Law Commission (1993,n.18) interprets 'advance directives' as anticipatory decisions, and distinguishes them from a living will which they define as 'an advance directive which is concerned with the refusal of life-sustaining procedures in the event of a terminal illness.' But in both the UK and the US the moral justification for advance directives is the promotion of individual autonomy and whilst they may specify options to receive certain forms of therapy, in the public mind and in most of the arguments designed to promote them, they are associated with opportunities to refuse therapy in the face of perceived fear of over-treatment.

Development of Advance Directives

The modern origins of the development of advance directives is in March 1976 when the New Jersey Supreme Court ruled that the 'right of privacy' permitted termination of therapy in the case of Karen Quinlan, a young women in a PVS whose parents successfully petitioned the courts for the withdrawal of ventilatory support. When ventilation was withdrawn Ms. Quinlan was able to breathe unaided and remained in a PVS until her death several years later. The *Quinlan* ruling initiated a new era in treatment abatement which recognised an ethical requirement to limit therapy. It established in law that there is a point beyond which a doctor has no duty to proceed with a treatment that is useless. The *Quinlan* decision was followed within seven months by the Californian Natural Death Act and similar legislation in several other states, according to which patients, under certain stringently defined conditions, could forego life-prolonging therapy. (Keene, 1978, Lamb, 1987) During the next ten years an increasing number of American court's decisions acknowledged that autonomous patients may refuse therapy on the legal grounds of 'privacy' - even when refusal may result in death. The developing case law also reveals that an adult's right to refuse therapy may be upheld even though he or she has lost the capacity to make such a decision.

In 1985 attention focused on the removal of life-sustaining nutrition and hydration when the New Jersey Supreme Court ruled that technological means of administering nutrition and hydration (a nasogastric tube) could be removed from a non-autonomous patient, Claire Conroy, an 84 year old woman with serious mental impairment and a limited life expectancy, on the authorization of a surrogate. That same year saw considerable legislation concerning advance directives, living wills and Natural Death Acts with statements on nutrition and hydration. At present some 40 states and the District of Columbia have legislation on advance directives which allow for the removal of 'medical treatment'. In some states, for example Maryland, a living will is restricted to terminal conditions, whilst arrangements for durable powers of health attorney are not so restricted. Further steps which firmly established the legal basis of advance directives include the Patient Self-Determination Act which, from 1 December, 1991, tied Medicare and Medicaid reimbursement for hospital and nursing homes to the provision of information about the use of living wills and advance directives. Hospitals and nursing homes which do not have a system in place for educating patients and staff about advance planning are excluded from Medicare and Medicaid funding. This clearly extends the scope of patient refusal and has been widely proclaimed as a benefit to the taxpayer. Ironically there are no provisions for the extension of health-care funding for those whose capacity for choice is restricted in the face of under-provision of health-care.

In Denmark advance directives are operative, after a law came into force in September, 1992, that requires doctors to check on a central register whether terminally ill patients have made one. On the Danish model patients must register with a central authority and submit a three-part form specifying categories of impairment for which an advance directive regarding therapy abatement could be implemented. Only the first category of impairment is legally binding; that the patient would not wish to receive life-prolonging treatment if he/she was 'irrevocably in the process of dying'. 'Dying' is then defined as the certainty that death will occur in days or weeks despite therapy. Examples such as terminal cancer, heart failure, and kidney failure are cited. However, in the other categories directives to forego therapy, which would leave the patient in a severe state of disability, and wishes for accelerated death as a side-effect of pain-killing drugs, could be overridden after careful consideration by two responsible physicians. One statement, nevertheless, runs close to euthanasia: it records a desire not to undergo treatment to prolong life if 'illness, advanced decrepitude, senile decay, accident, heart problems, or similar situations have led to a situation of such severe invalidity that [he or she] would permanently be incapable of taking care of [himself or herself] physically and mentally'. (Dolley, 1993) Six months after the register was established only forty inquiries had been made. At present, over 65,000 Danes have registered out of a population of 3.9 million. (Holm, 1994) Criticism of the scheme has come from the Danish Medical Association who argue that the informal nature of the procedure does not ensure that the person in question is competent to make a decision of this kind. They also complain that there is ambiguity in the expression 'irreversibly dying', and that the procedures for checking if a specific patient is registered are time-consuming, especially for emergency room physicians. (Holm, 1994)

A strong expression of patient autonomy is found in the Medical Treatment Act, 1988, of Victoria, Australia, which enables a patient to refuse therapy on the basis of a certificate signed by a competent person over the age of eighteen who is under no compulsion and inducement and is fully informed as to the consequences of refusal. This act also introduced the concept of 'medical trespass' which is committed by a medical practitioner who knowingly treats contrary to the provision of a certificate. The Act has no provisions for a doctor or nurse's conscience clause, and it makes no distinction between terminal and other illnesses: the right to refuse treatment is unqualified.

Although living wills have not been widely discussed in the UK until recently, there are signs of public interest in them. In 1988 the Age Concern Institute of Gerontology published a report under the title, 'The Living Will, Consent to Treatment at the End of Life' which generated interest in the subject. In 1993 two Private Members Bills were introduced in Parliament on living wills, but were unsuccessful. The Voluntary Euthanasia Society - EXIT - claim that they issue about 20,000 living wills each year. In November 1992 the BMA issued a statement supporting living wills. It endorsed advance directives and health-care proxies, and drew attention to the advisability of renewing their terms every five years. The Terence Higgins Trust devised a living will form in October 1992 in cooperation with the Centre of Medical Law and Ethics at Kings College London. This particular form, of which 10,000 copies had been distributed between 1992 and 1994, was specifically designed in the interests of people with HIV and AIDS. As a precaution this living will includes a statement which stresses that it is not a substitute for discussion with a doctor. Many solicitors in the UK are said to be preparing living wills on their clients instructions. The BMA reported to the House of Lords Select Committee on Medical Ethics (1994:39) on an 'upsurge in public interest,' but did not favour legislation to enforce advance directives. The same Committee heard evidence from Scottish Action on Dementia (SAD) who said that 'there would not be the current interest in and demand for living wills in the United Kingdom if current codes of professional ethics were meeting peoples needs.' (*ibid*:39) SAD also complained that doctors in the UK displayed little respect for patients autonomy but they believed that advance directives could redress this situation. A spokesperson from the Royal College of Nursing expressed concern over the risks of legally enforced advance directives on the grounds that they might lead to 'defensive practices' but in general supported advance directives as a measure to secure prospective autonomy. Thus 'many people...are not necessarily afraid of death, but are afraid of the manner of death... For them writing a living will gives them comfort, not least because they feel they are able to continue to have control and autonomy in their lives, even at a time when they can no longer exercise that autonomy directly.' (*ibid*:39) Further support was expressed by the Alzheimer's Disease Society in a written memorandum to the House of Lords Select Committee on Medical Ethics, which drew a distinction between advance directives and proposals to decriminalise euthanasia. The Patient's Association in the United Kingdom also declared support for advance directives, saying that 'a general indication of a patient's wishes made and recorded formally, should relieve the doctor of the responsibility of acting without consent.' (*ibid*:40) It was also noted that an advance directive would relieve the family of the anxiety bound up with taking difficult decisions and would avoid disputes of the sort which have arisen in recent AIDS cases between the wishes of the family and those of the partner.

There has been little public discussion of health-care agents in England and Wales. At common law no one may consent to treatment on behalf of an incapable patient. Any weight given to the views of a health-care agent will, for the present, be determined by the patient's doctor. However, the Law Commission in England has recommended a statutory framework for health-care agents, which are referred to as 'medical treatment attorneys.' The Mental Health and Disability Sub-Committee of the Law Society in the UK favour a combination of advance directives and proxy decision-makers:

> This combination would have the advantage of setting down the person's wishes on a legal document, while also appointing someone to ensure those wishes are enforced, as well as being able to make related decisions which may not have been clearly specified in the advance directive. (Evidence to the House of Lords Select Committee on Medical Ethics, 1994:45).

Legal and medical opinion in the UK appears to be moving in favour of proxy arrangements. Campaigns are already under way to provide information regarding their pros and cons. Professor Ian Kennedy, a society approves. It can be an arena of abuse and forced marriages are possible by means of blackmail or fear of violence. But we still support and cherish the institution of marriage whilst seeking to minimise abuse. So, she says, the same can be said of euthanasia in the Netherlands. The analogy has one fundamental limitation: abuse of the voluntary principle in marriage can always be rectified by annulment and divorce giving the victims a possibility of building a new life; with euthanasia there is no remedy and no life to rebuild.

Opponents of Dutch medical practice might argue that the Netherlands have begun a slippery slope which started with a justification of euthanasia strictly on the explicit request of a patient and then developed into a justification of non-requested deaths. It is, however, hard to establish a slippery slope in this instance as there is no hard data on the starting point. Such data could be provided if a survey of accelerated deaths had been conducted ten years ago. Nevertheless, a process appears to be under way whereby the justification of euthanasia was extended from an appeal to patient autonomy to an appeal to the doctor's moral beliefs. It might be noted that in the Netherlands, despite the alleged importance attributed to patient autonomy, it is often trumped by medical wisdom; two thirds of euthanasia requests are rejected by doctors (Deldon Loes, 1993). This would suggest that a criterion other than autonomy is being used.

Battin points out that the euthanasia programme in the Netherlands has emerged against a background of greater equality of access to healthcare than is available in the US in a society that is more tolerant of its composite social groups. There is less likelihood of abuse, she maintains, than in the US. Nevertheless, two lessons can be learnt from the Netherlands' experiment. First, in a climate in which there is profit in the elimination of unwanted people, and a significant proportion of influential people (particularly doctors) are committed to a programme of killing, then further steps down a slippery slope towards the killing of those who do not want to die is highly probable. (Lamb, 1988) Second, the Netherlands' experiment reveals how easy a society's commitment to individual autonomy can be surrendered once judgements like 'futility', 'unbearable', 'medically inappropriate', and that 'life has been ... given up' are regarded as purely clinical matters unrelated to moral discourse.

III Advance Directives and Living Wills

Introduction

The question addressed by proponents of living wills is the right to direct treatment during the end stages of one's life, especially when a stage is reached where one is no longer competent to make a rational decision. The media as well as the writings of many bioethicists have reported widespread fear of painful death in institutional isolation in circumstances where the disease process has severely limited the ability to make decisions concerning treatment options. A living will is a document upon which individuals can indicate in advance a preference not to be given various forms of therapy to prolong life. Living wills can also give directions for refusing specific forms of therapy, including blood transfusions, CPR, chemotherapy, renal dialysis, various intubations, ventilators, and nutrition and hydration. Many caring and compassionate institutions and individuals have supported them as a means of providing a patient with some means of control over his or her death, and extend personal autonomy into areas where the capacity to act autonomously is lost. Yet whilst the living will conveys a written expression of a person's desires it is difficult to imagine and comprehensively list all possible medical contingencies. Thus living wills are of limited value. Their precise interpretation may require further discussion with a doctor at a time when treatment decisions are to be taken. Hence in some American states durable powers of attorney statutes have emerged, whereby one can appoint an agent to act for oneself at any time after loss of the capacity for self-determination. In this respect the health-care power of attorney is a device to enable the patient to tell the doctor who the surrogate or proxy should be. Their legal force is stronger than living wills and in some states in the US the appointed agent's authority may overrule objections from family members. Taken together, 'living wills' or 'health-care powers of attorney' are known as 'advance directives.' Legal opinion in the UK, where laws are being considered to give further living wills and Natural Death Acts with statements on nutrition and hydration. At present some 40 states and the District of Columbia have legislation on advance directives which allow for the removal of 'medical treatment'. In some states, for example Maryland, a living will is restricted to terminal conditions, whilst arrangements for durable powers of health attorney are not so restricted. Further steps which firmly established the legal basis of advance directives include the Patient Self-Determination Act which, from 1 December, 1991, tied Medicare and Medicaid reimbursement for hospital and nursing homes to the provision of information about the use of living wills and advance directives. Hospitals and nursing homes which do not have a system in place for educating patients and staff about advance planning are excluded from Medicare and Medicaid funding. This clearly extends the scope of patient refusal and has been widely proclaimed as a benefit to the taxpayer. Ironically there are no provisions for the extension of health-care funding for those whose capacity for choice is restricted in the face of under-provision of health-care.

In Denmark advance directives are operative, after a law came into force in September, 1992, that requires doctors to check on a central register whether terminally ill patients have made one. On the Danish model patients must register with a central authority and submit a three-part form specifying categories of impairment for which an advance directive regarding therapy abatement could be implemented. Only the first category of impairment is legally binding; that the patient would not wish to receive life-prolonging treatment if he/she was 'irrevocably in the process of dying'. 'Dying' is then defined as the certainty that death will occur in days or weeks despite therapy. Examples such as terminal cancer, heart failure, and kidney failure are cited. However, in the other categories directives to forego therapy, which would leave the patient in a severe state of disability, and wishes for accelerated death as a side-effect of pain-killing drugs, could be overridden after careful consideration by two responsible physicians. One statement, nevertheless, runs close to euthanasia: it records a desire not to undergo treatment to prolong life if 'illness, advanced decrepitude, senile decay, accident, heart problems, or similar situations have led to a situation of such severe invalidity that [he or she] would permanently be incapable of taking care of [himself or herself] physically and mentally'. (Dolley, 1993) Six months after the register was established only forty inquiries had been made. At present, over 65,000 Danes have registered out of a population of 3.9 million. (Holm, 1994) Criticism of the scheme has come from the Danish Medical Association who argue that the informal recognition to advance directives, is slightly different to the US. In England the Law Commission (1993,n.18) interprets 'advance directives' as anticipatory decisions, and distinguishes them from a living will which they define as 'an advance directive which is concerned with the refusal of life-sustaining procedures in the event of a terminal illness.' But in both the UK and the US the moral justification for advance directives is the promotion of individual autonomy and whilst they may specify options to receive certain forms of therapy, in the public mind and in most of the arguments designed to promote them, they are associated with opportunities to refuse therapy in the face of perceived fear of over-treatment.

Development of Advance Directives

The modern origins of the development of advance directives is in March 1976 when the New Jersey Supreme Court ruled that the 'right of privacy' permitted termination of therapy in the case of Karen Quinlan, a young women in a PVS whose parents successfully petitioned the courts for the withdrawal of ventilatory support. When ventilation was withdrawn Ms. Quinlan was able to breathe unaided and remained in a PVS until her death several years later. The *Quinlan* ruling initiated a new era in treatment abatement which recognised an ethical requirement to limit therapy. It established in law that there is a point beyond which a doctor has no duty to proceed with a treatment that is useless. The *Quinlan* decision was followed within seven months by the Californian Natural Death Act and similar legislation in several other states, according to which patients, under certain stringently defined conditions, could forego life-prolonging therapy. (Keene, 1978, Lamb, 1987) During the next ten years an increasing number of American court's decisions acknowledged that autonomous patients may refuse therapy on the legal grounds of 'privacy' - even when refusal may result in death. The developing case law also reveals that an adult's right to refuse therapy may be upheld even though he or she has lost the capacity to make such a decision.

In 1985 attention focused on the removal of life-sustaining nutrition and hydration when the New Jersey Supreme Court ruled that technological means of administering nutrition and hydration (a nasogastric tube) could be removed from a non-autonomous patient, Claire Conroy, an 84 year old woman with serious mental impairment and a limited life expectancy, on the authorization of a surrogate. That same year saw considerable legislation concerning advance directives, nature of the procedure does not ensure that the person in question is competent to make a decision of this kind. They also complain that there is ambiguity in the expression 'irreversibly dying', and that the procedures for checking if a specific patient is registered are time-consuming, especially for emergency room physicians. (Holm, 1994)

A strong expression of patient autonomy is found in the Medical Treatment Act, 1988, of Victoria, Australia, which enables a patient to refuse therapy on the basis of a certificate signed by a competent person over the age of eighteen who is under no compulsion and inducement and is fully informed as to the consequences of refusal. This act also introduced the concept of 'medical trespass' which is committed by a medical practitioner who knowingly treats contrary to the provision of a certificate. The Act has no provisions for a doctor or nurse's conscience clause, and it makes no distinction between terminal and other illnesses: the right to refuse treatment is unqualified.

Although living wills have not been widely discussed in the UK until recently, there are signs of public interest in them. In 1988 the Age Concern Institute of Gerontology published a report under the title, 'The Living Will, Consent to Treatment at the End of Life' which generated interest in the subject. In 1993 two Private Members Bills were introduced in Parliament on living wills, but were unsuccessful. The Voluntary Euthanasia Society - EXIT - claim that they issue about 20,000 living wills each year. In November 1992 the BMA issued a statement supporting living wills. It endorsed advance directives and health-care proxies, and drew attention to the advisability of renewing their terms every five years. The Terence Higgins Trust devised a living will form in October 1992 in cooperation with the Centre of Medical Law and Ethics at Kings College London. This particular form, of which 10,000 copies had been distributed between 1992 and 1994, was specifically designed in the interests of people with HIV and AIDS. As a precaution this living will includes a statement which stresses that it is not a substitute for discussion with a doctor. Many solicitors in the UK are said to be preparing living wills on their clients instructions. The BMA reported to the House of Lords Select Committee on Medical Ethics (1994:39) on an 'upsurge in public interest,' but did not favour legislation to enforce advance directives. The same Committee heard evidence from Scottish Action on Dementia (SAD) who said that 'there would not be the current interest in and demand for living wills in the United Kingdom if current codes of professional ethics were meeting peoples needs.' (*ibid*:39) SAD also complained that doctors in the UK displayed little respect for patients autonomy but they believed that advance directives could redress this situation. A spokesperson from the Royal College of Nursing expressed concern over the risks of legally enforced advance directives on the grounds that they might lead to 'defensive practices' but in general supported advance directives as a measure to secure prospective autonomy. Thus 'many people...are not necessarily afraid of death, but are afraid of the manner of death... For them writing a living will gives them comfort, not least because they feel they are able to continue to have control and autonomy in their lives, even at a time when they can no longer exercise that autonomy directly.' (*ibid*:39) Further support was expressed by the Alzheimer's Disease Society in a written memorandum to the House of Lords Select Committee on Medical Ethics, which drew a distinction between advance directives and proposals to decriminalise euthanasia. The Patient's Association in the United Kingdom also declared support for advance directives, saying that 'a general indication of a patient's wishes made and recorded formally, should relieve the doctor of the responsibility of acting without consent.' (*ibid*:40) It was also noted that an advance directive would relieve the family of the anxiety bound up with taking difficult decisions and would avoid disputes of the sort which have arisen in recent AIDS cases between the wishes of the family and those of the partner.

There has been little public discussion of health-care agents in England and Wales. At common law no one may consent to treatment on behalf of an incapable patient. Any weight given to the views of a health-care agent will, for the present, be determined by the patient's doctor. However, the Law Commission in England has recommended a statutory framework for health-care agents, which are referred to as 'medical treatment attorneys.' The Mental Health and Disability Sub-Committee of the Law Society in the UK favour a combination of advance directives and proxy decision-makers:

> This combination would have the advantage of setting down the person's wishes on a legal document, while also appointing someone to ensure those wishes are enforced, as well as being able to make related decisions which may not have been clearly specified in the advance directive. (Evidence to the House of Lords Select Committee on Medical Ethics, 1994:45).

Legal and medical opinion in the UK appears to be moving in favour of proxy arrangements. Campaigns are already under way to provide information regarding their pros and cons. Professor Ian Kennedy, a supporter of proxy arrangements for post-competent patients, has nevertheless expressed certain reservations with the proposal to give them statutory backing. In an interview reported in *The Observer*, 26 February, 1995, he said that; 'The fundamental problem is that the proxy idea is very much a middle-class solution. Many people do not have someone who is rational enough to stand up for their interests when dealing with doctors and other health-care workers. But it is better than nothing. The current law is that no one can consent or refuse treatment on behalf of another adult'. It should be stressed that class or lack of education will not provide such a problem when devising ways for a patient to forego expensive life-prolonging health-care. Few members of the lower-classes, in a grossly underfunded health-service, see compulsory over-treatment as a threat to their dignity.

Proposed Benefits of Advance Directives

There appears to be widespread support for living wills and advance directives among bioethicists, especially for prior decisions concerning future incompetency. Their moral and legal basis is the autonomy interest in avoiding bodily intrusions. Their alleged benefits are bound up with a sense of control over future decisions regarding the end points of life. According to Norman L. Cantor, an architect of U.S. legislation supporting advance directives:

> The potential benefits of an advance directive are plain. Not only can persons prospectively promote personal values and concepts of dignity, but the ultimate decision makers on behalf of the incompetent patient can receive crucial guidance. An advance directive can guide health-care providers as to the agent to be responsible for decision-making, as to substantive wishes of the declarant regarding care, or both. A health-care agent or, in the absence of a designated agent, any person acting as formal or informal guardian of the incompetent patient also can receive guidance as to the wishes of the patient. This guidance might mitigate the anxiety, uncertainty, or conflicts sometimes surrounding terminal decisions on behalf of incompetent patients. (Cantor, 1993:23)

For Cantor the ultimate case for advance directives is their propensity to 'exercise prospective autonomy.' (*ibid*:23) This objective, as we shall later see, is not without related problems.

John F. Robertson (1991:6) outlines what appear to be the two foremost benefits of living wills:

1. The living will thus empowers people, by extending the scope of personal autonomy to situations in which autonomy cannot be directly exercised.

2. ...living wills, if specific enough, provide a worthwhile rule for non-treatment decisions that *appears* to respect autonomy without compromising respect for incompetent patients.

They are certainly more reliable than recollections of a patient's known wishes.

Problems with Advance Directives

Yet despite the enthusiasm shown by bioethicists, governments and the media, advance directives and living wills have not proved as popular with the general public as anticipated. In 1988, less than 10% of the US population had either a living will or a durable power of attorney (Emanuel and Emanuel, 1989) whilst a 1988 USA survey revealed 90% of respondents had a positive attitude to advance directives, less than one in ten had completed one. Another study revealed only 21% of the population of very seriously ill hospitalized patients had been reported to have signed advance directives (Lynn and Teno, 1993). Even after the publicity surrounding *Cruzan* (1990) and the Patient's Self Determination Act 1991, only 20% of US patients made use of advance directives. (Emanuel and Emanuel, 1993) Doctors are often sceptical of the value of living wills, expressing criticism of their vagueness and inappropriateness during the clinical management of patient care. An advance directive is critically dependent upon a prognosis. To activate a directive specifying selective abatement in the event of a terminal condition it may be required that a doctor confirms no hope of recovery, or imminent death, or a state of disability. But a prognosis is not an expression of certitude; it is at best a guess based on known possibilities.

The boundaries of acceptable disability are also difficult to capture in a document. As a spokesperson for CARE pointed out to the House of Lords Select Committee on Medical Ethics: (1994:41) 'disabled individuals are commonly more satisfied with their life than able-bodied people would expect to be with the same disability. The healthy do not choose in the same way as the sick.' Evidence is also growing of the ineffectiveness of advance directives in actually assuring patient autonomy. It has become apparent that few patients actually want to manage their own dying, but prefer to leave decisions to close relatives. A survey conducted among nursing personnel in 1992 at the University of Maryland Medical System (Silverman *et al*, 1994) indicated concern that inquiries about advance directives can deliver a mixed message concerning prognosis and treatment. Nurses reported that even raising the issue of advance directives could cause anxiety to patients and their families and that such inquiries were particularly threatening to patients facing surgery. Patients frequently interpreted a request to discuss advance directives, which is legally required under the Patient Self Determination Act, as a concealed hint that something was wrong. Generally, the nurses in Silverman *et al's* survey found that patients had little interest in discussing advance directives. This reluctance to issue advance directives may be put down to a refusal to confront one's own mortality, argues Cantor, (1993:34) who admits that 'best estimates are that only fifteen to twenty five percent of adults have signed a living will, though the percentage is higher for persons over the age of sixty four.' It may also indicate that the perceived fear of overtreatment has been exaggerated.

A number of recently conducted surveys on the role of advance directives in securing autonomous decision-making and improved doctor-patient communication indicate that they may not be as effective as predicted. Whilst studies have indicated that up to 28% of AIDS patients have taken out advance directives (Teno, *et al*, 1994:23) there are indications that they are having little effect upon treatment decisions for other seriously ill patients. A survey by J. Virmani, L. J. Schneiderman and R. M. Kaplan (1994) interviewed 115 seriously ill cancer patients and 22 of their doctors on various aspects of the application of the advance directives they had executed. The results were then compared with the treatment of patients who had not executed them. The overall results indicated that 'despite public enthusiasm for the use of advance directives and great efforts to promote them', there was 'little evidence that these documents are associated with enhanced communication between patients and physicians about end-of-life treatment decisions'. (Virmani *et al*, 1994:909) It was found that doctors, for the most part were unaware of their patient's advance directives, and whilst those with advance directives were marginally more likely, than those without them, to report discussions about end-of-life decisions, only 34 (30%) out of the 115 claimed to have engaged in discussions about treatment decisions. The report noted that 'overall communication on these matters between physicians and patients seems to be low'. (Virmani *et al*, 1994:913)

This absence of communication suggests that doctors are not taking the initiative in raising the subject of advance directives with their patients. However, other surveys indicate that despite advance directives doctors still project their own preferences into treatment. (Schneiderman *et al*, 1993)

Further evidence of the practical ineffectiveness of advance directives is seen in a survey carried out by SUPPORT (Study to Understand Prognosis and Preferences for Outcomes and Risks of Treatment), which found 'no significant association between the existence of advance directives and decisions about resuscitation'. (Teno *et al*, 1994:26) This survey was conducted among 3058 seriously ill patients in an American hospital with a view to finding out the effects of advance directives on decisions regarding resuscitation. The findings are conclusive: 'Patients who had advance directives were no more likely than other patients to prefer to forego resuscitation.....advance directives were irrelevant to decision-making.....Advance directives had no clinically important effect on decision-making concerning resuscitation among the seriously ill patients in SUPPORT'. (Teno *et al*, 1994:27) The survey found only a mere 1% increase in reports of having an advance directive leading to having a discussion with a physician. And this, said the report, 'might well arise from a biased recollection - those who organise their lives enough to write advance directives might also remember talking to their physicians'. (*ibid*:27) The report concluded that 'these findings fail to support the widespread public and professional enthusiasm for advance directives'. (*ibid*:27)

In a commentary on the SUPPORT survey Dan W. Brock (1994) drew some interesting conclusions. He suggested that 'the still widespread assumption that dying patients are over-treated may be wrong'. (Brock, 1994:59) He also raised an important question about the role of advance directives: are they, he asked, devices to prevent over-treatment or are they intended to limit costs of patient care? As evidence suggests that they have no effect on the former what is their effect on the latter? It would seem that advance directives are ineffective here also, and Brock cites surveys which indicate that advance directives have led, in some instances, to escalating costs. Whilst savings were widely predicted and expected, they have failed to materialise. Nevertheless, as Brock notes, there is a likelihood that despite their ineffectiveness regarding treatment decisions, savings in health-care expenditure may come from advance directives which express a wish not to be hospitalised.

There are expressed fears that medical care will be adversely affected if an advance directive is signed, and that legislation empowering them is merely a gimmick in order to legitimise even further rationing of health-care. These objections are reinforced by the tendency of living will exponents to bait their appeal to autonomy with utilitarian benefits. As Cantor (1993:29) says:

> Another utilitarian benefit is the saving of public resources. That is, widespread use of implementations of advance directives might well result in reduced resort to expensive life-preserving medical machinery. This could be an incidental public benefit flowing from the upholding of future-orientated autonomy. I am not contending that these general public benefits provide a morally sufficient basis for enforcing advance directives. They do, however, reinforce the self-determination arguments for upholding a competent person's advance directive.

Although Cantor is clear that the moral foundation for advance directives is prospective autonomy, a greater emphasis on the utilitarian benefits is to be expected from budget restrained administrators and cost-conscious governments. Those already experiencing the ill-effects of budgetary restraints on health-care provisions will not be persuaded by these arguments that it is in their interests to further reduce their access to expensive life-preserving machinery.

There is evidence, too, that the element of doctor-patient trust, which is essential to the success of an advance directive, is breaking down. This can be seen in the increasing rate of law suits over advance directives and the anonymous context in which health-care is provided. In this respect advance directives reveal their paradoxical nature; they can only guarantee autonomy in the context of complete trust between doctor and patient, but the purported rationale behind the advance directive is to provide safeguards for autonomy when trust is lacking because of the anonymous situation in which health-care is provided. Some advocates of advance directives have insisted that an advance directive is not a substitute for decision-making in the context of detailed consultations between doctor and patient. (See Cantor, 1993) Although critics have warned that a document would tend to replace dialogue the BMA have argued that advance directives would actually enable dialogue between doctor and patient. In this respect the BMA's position is hopelessly unrealistic and is based upon a notion of close doctor-patient consultation which may have existed for a minority of middle to upper class families in the early decades of this century, but more likely a feature of the cinema's portrayal of the family doctor who is always on hand for advice, and usually marries the eldest daughter. Given the amount of time a busy doctor in an underfunded health service can spend with each patient it is likely that an advance directive, drawn up by some other professional agency, will be fed into the computer and one day activated without a lengthy period of doctor-patient consultation. Thus advance directives could spawn an industry of advisors who will assist healthy people to draw up increasingly complex documents which attempt to deal with every possible medical contingency. On a more positive note, well-drafted advance directives would be highly beneficial in a flourishing system of health-care teams where decisions are collectively taken, with consultation covering a broad range of moral and religious views.

There are practical problems in determining whether or not the directive represents what a patient would actually want. For example, new highly beneficial therapy may be developed which the patient was unaware of at the time of signing the directive. A treatment which once had a bad reputation, was highly experimental with risks of unpleasant side-effects and listed among therapies to be withheld, may evolve into a safe routine therapy without the patient's awareness. Fears have also been expressed that an advance directive might be formulated without the patient actually appreciating what it would be like to actually experience the conditions under which the treatment might be offered. There are major resource problems involved in implementing mechanisms for the revision of advance directives. How often should they be revised? As a disease process develops there is considerable scope for revision of former beliefs and attitudes. Likewise a greater understanding of an ability to cope with disability may change an earlier perspective. The resources required to record such changes within a legalistic framework could be immense. A further problem is that the assumptions on which an advance directive is based might not be clearly translated into practice. A patient may wish to forego cardiopulmonary resuscitation (CPR) on the assumption that declining CPR is appropriate when her overall condition has deteriorated to the point where CPR is futile and she will not survive the attempt. But she might not wish to forego CPR which could be initiated after cardiac arrest in response to a medical procedure or reaction to a drug, in circumstances where recovery without impairment is highly probable. These areas of uncertainty could provide grounds for overriding an advanced directive.

Among the practical problems in devising advance directives as a means of securing autonomy is that the document would require mention of an infinite number of hypothetical facts and circumstances which would govern decision-making, as well as changes in a person's attitude towards death and incapacity. Even if all this were not recorded in a document, so the objection runs, it would be unfair to expect the proxy or health-care agent to examine every contingency. Cantor (1993) insists that this objection can be contained. Although it is not possible to specify every contingent prospective medical state, some general principles can be expressed in advance, such as religious objections to blood transfusions, or aversion to being permanently unconscious. Nevertheless, a full and effective use of advance directives requires a level of sophistication and involvement by patients or their surrogates which is far from reality. The inability of many patients to comprehend a prognosis and therapy options has been well-documented in several surveys. In a study of procedures for evaluating informed consent Allan Templeton (1995:292) refers to a study of patients undergoing neurosurgery who, despite instructions by a neurosurgeon and a clinical nurse specialist, only retained 50% of information given to them about operative risks and possible outcomes. Templeton also referred to studies in various countries which reveal poor retention of information, patients signing consent forms without understanding them and, in some cases, without even reading them. 'Despite these and other findings,' says Templeton, (*ibid*:292) 'doctors continue to derive unreasonable reassurance from a signed consent form.'

The lesson to be learnt from studies of well-established practices for eliciting informed consent is that large sections of the population may require considerable assistance in drafting health-care plans. Information on treatment options would have to cater for a public with limited powers of comprehension. For example, the average adult reading age in the UK is that of a ten year old child. In a study of advance directives among the elderly in the USA, Dallas M. High (1993) pointed out that educational level and ethnic background played a significant role. Whilst 35% of whites in the study had taken out living wills only 2% of blacks had done so. Most studies confirm that advance directives are preferred by well-educated white people. This is not surprising, as they belong to a group who receive most care, counselling and attention, from their doctors.

Can we really expect the poor, the unemployed and undereducated to believe that such mechanisms and laws are there to protect them from over-treatment? For many people the promotion of advance directives is perceived as a gimmick to reduce health-care costs, not as a means of extending their scope for self-determination. Greg A. Sachs (1994:15) notes this negative aspect and points out that: 'Uninsured patients who only get through private hospital doors when they are too sick to be transferred to a city or county hospital are unlikely to feel "empowered" by the opportunity to fill out a directive enabling them to forego treatment.' Nevertheless, Sachs and other proponents of advance directives urge further intervention to increase their use as vehicles for future health-care planning. This raises the question whether more intervention is required to promote advance directives or whether, in the light of the criticisms that have been made of them, we should recognise their limitations for public policy?

To date interventions to promote advance directives have not been very successful. Education brochures, physician-initiated counselling and widespread media alarms about over-treatment have not altered the fact that the majority of people do not take out advance directives. (See Teno, Nelson, and Lynn, 1994) Efforts have been promoted to eliminate potential bias in the means of communicating health-care options, and undoubtedly further efforts at refinement could continue. Robert Allan Pearlman (1994:26) suggests that:

> If use of advance directives remains low after further refinements and efficacy trials, then interventions could focus on overcoming barriers to advance care planning. Educational interventions could target patients; reimbursements could promote physician involvement. A review of recent changes in social practices would help determine what motivates people to desire these changes... The ability of experts and marketing to influence our tastes, desires and aspirations could also be channelled to promote advance directives. Focus groups could uncover motivations, barriers, and acceptable strategies, as well as measure and evaluate the influence of hope, uncertainty about the future, and attitudes, and attitudes towards risk.

These measures may very well result in an increased public acceptance of advance directives, but the reliance upon techniques of attitude formation and manipulation raise questions concerning enhanced patient autonomy as the ethical rationale of advance health-care planning.

If advance directives do not deliver an autonomous choice does the solution lie in intervention designed to encourage greater involvement or is there a deeper problem? One of the criticisms highlighted here (and again in chapter VIII) is with the notion of autonomous choice which health-care documents are designed to promote. The mechanisms designed to promote autonomy in a health-care setting rest on an Enlightenment view of the self which exists in a state of detachment from other interests and selves, and seeks satisfaction in the maximisation of its preferences. This is clearly a metaphysical notion of the self, which crudely represents a market orientation towards social life, where patients are consumers and health-care professionals are seen as suppliers of merchandise. There are, however, alternative views of the self which are not based on a level of detachment associated with an individual maximisation of preferences but seek satisfaction in social relationships. The reduction of selfhood to an ensemble of consumer relations is not easily attained in a health-care setting. A completed document may not fulfil the requirements for self-determination. Respect for autonomy is not something that is initiated in a hospital; it is bound up with a life-time of free actions. Whilst appeal to the principle of self-determination has considerable moral merit, its isolation from the broader context of autonomous self-fulfilment - which has no reality for the vast majority of people - renders it formal and meaningless in the context of health-care.

Advance Directives and Euthanasia

One major ethical problem with advance directives concerns the potential for abuse, in the sense that many proponents of euthanasia (both voluntary and non-voluntary) support them as part of a strategy to relax existing prohibitions on euthanasia. Some pro-euthanasia pressure groups see no distinction between therapy abatement and euthanasia and would welcome an extension of therapy abatement to include 'merciful release' or physician-assisted dying.

To appreciate the potential for the abuse of advance directives it is necessary to examine some of the earliest proposals for living wills where therapy abatement was not so clearly separated from directives to kill. The earliest proponent appears to be Luis Kutner, a Chicago attorney who drafted a living will in the 1930's in response to 'barbaric' medical treatment inflicted against the protests of a dying friend. (Weir, 1990:181) The document was circulated and the first person to sign it was Bishop Fulton Sheen. The second was Errol Flynn. In the 1960's the document was taken up by the United States Euthanasia Education

Council. In 1969 Kutner published a paper in *The Indiana Law Journal* under the title 'Due Process of Euthanasia: Living Will, A Proposal'. Although Kutner did not openly advocate euthanasia in his paper it was clear that this was what he had in mind. In his concluding remarks he said, 'as of now a doctor cannot be directed to act affirmatively to terminate a patient's life', (*ibid*:553).

In recent years there has been a general shift towards a limited 'right-to-die' in the USA as well as several European countries. It is bound up with a relaxation of suicide laws and a general acceptance of the right to forego life-prolonging therapy, limited perhaps to obligations on others not to interfere with a patient's choice. Strictly speaking there is an emerging right to be left to die, rather than a right to die. This is the ultimate rationale of advance directives. So what more can pro-euthanasia and right-to-die movements want? The answer, so it would appear, is a legal framework in which medical assistance can be provided in putting into effect a choice in favour of death. With few exceptions the courts and health-care organisations have resisted this step.

The current debate over advance directives has taken place in the context of a moral panic, akin to the premature burial panic of the late nineteenth century. In this case concern is with over-treatment and extended life treatment rather than under treatment and hastily diagnosed death. Advance directives have been embraced by euthanasia enthusiasts, advocates of medical cost-containment, and civil libertarians anxious to extend the scope of patient autonomy. Not all of these supporters of advance directives share the same moral premises. Cantor, (1993) a prominent advocate of advance directives, argues that properly formulated advance directives are the answer to a morally questionable acceptance of euthanasia. Yet in many of the arguments put forward in favour of advance directives it is not always clear whether the goal is prospective autonomy, euthanasia or medical cost-containment. Exponents of all three positions may very well appeal to concepts of personal freedom, dignity, choice, and the rights of the individual. The recent Report of the House of Lords Select Committee on Medical Ethics (1994), which concluded in support of the legal enhancement of advance directives, but condemned euthanasia, nevertheless confused arguments for medical cost-containment with arguments for giving an individual greater control over therapy options. The Committee expressed concern that advances in medical technology had led to situations where patients could live longer, but that in some cases this raised questions whether such treatment was a benefit or a burden to the patient.

As medicine has overcome many life-threatening conditions more and more of the population are surviving longer and facing the chronic degenerative conditions which old age may bring. The social implications of this are enormous, since the care adequately for the resulting large numbers of sick and elderly patients is difficult and costly. (House of Lords Select Committee on Medical Ethics, 1994:7)

These remarks reveal how easily an ethical defence of autonomous therapy refusal can be converted to a solution to the problems of medical cost-containment. This kind of argument has been constantly repeated throughout the debate on advance directives with the result that the validity of an autonomous decision is in danger of being determined by the distributors of funds in the health-care market.

The fear that, once legalised, advance directives concerning treatment abatement may lead to a more permissive attitude towards euthanasia explains much of the pro-life opposition to them. In a written Memorandum to the House of Lords Select Committee on Medical Ethics (1994:67) the Christian Medical Fellowship noted how 'the language of advance directives reinforces negative images of disability and disease and feeds the patient's fears'. In giving expression to these fears opponents of euthanasia have been accused of adopting doctrinaire attitudes in favour of the curtailment of patient autonomy. Where possible pro-lifers have secured restrictive amendments to Natural Death Acts and Living Will legislation, which have been accepted by proponents of a more radical position in the belief that these amendments can be changed with 'clean up' legislation at a later time. (Weir 1990:197) In this context slippery slope predictions from pro-lifers have considerable significance. Proposals were put forward by the Hemlock Society of the USA for two advance directives not limited to the criteria for therapy abatement. The first is a 'Request for Help in Dying' which calls for acceleration of one's dying in the event of terminal illness; the second is a 'Request for Help in Dying by Proxy', which is a written directive for securing a physician's help by intentionally killing the patient.

The Hemlock Society has also tried, so far unsuccessfully, to promote a Humane and Dignified Death Act, as a substantial modification of existing Natural Death Acts. Its most controversial clause is an advance directive calling for a physician to 'administer 'aid in dying' in a humane and dignified manner'. The Hemlock Society interpret the expression 'aid-in-dying' as any medical procedure that will 'swiftly, painlessly and humanely terminate the life of the qualified patient'. This would include the use of a lethal injection or lethal overdose. If accepted the proposal for an 'aid-in-dying' would not only legitimise euthanasia; it would incorporate a legal obligation to kill. It would initiate a new departure in defensive medicine: by granting immunity from civil or criminal liability to those who 'humanely terminate the life of a qualified patient', but giving no protection to those who act in the belief that it is in the patient's best interest to provide maximum care, a situation could arise where erring on the side of death would be the safest course in any questionable situation.

In November, 1991 voters in Washington were given a chance to express a preference over Initiative Measure No.119 following a petition organised by Citizens for Death With Dignity containing 223,000 signatures of registered voters. It was defeated. But if passed Initiative 119 would have amended Washington's 1979 'Natural Death Act' to the 'Death With Dignity Act'. The initiative proposed a loosening of the definition of 'terminal condition' to include PVS patients, and provided the option of a voluntary 'aid-in-dying' as 'aid in the form of a medical service, provided in person by a physician, that will end the life of a conscious and mentally competent qualified patient in a dignified, painless and humane manner'. Opponents of Initiative 119 contended that the proposal would make it legal for doctors to administer a lethal dose on request.

The 'aid-in-dying' initiative was tried again in the State of California on the third of November, 1992, in a proposal for a 'Death With Dignity Act'. Proposition 161 had stricter safeguards than Washington's Initiative 119. The Californian proposal stressed that directives cannot be executed by doctors or nurses unless one of the two required witnesses is a patient advocate or ombudsman appointed by the state for that purpose. Quite obviously these 'safeguards' can be included and, as many pro- euthanasia proponents point out, amended with clean-up legislation sometime later. Nevertheless, despite a strong pro-death movement, in a state in which children can be legally executed, the Californian Death With Dignity Act was defeated by a 54 to 46 majority. Had it been enacted it would have legitimised euthanasia.

Following the Washington and California initiatives for physician assisted suicide was a less extreme proposal sponsored by the 'Oregon Right to Die' movement in 1994 which was designed to permit 'adults to request and obtain prescriptions from doctors to end their life.' Thus on 8 November, 1994, the voters in the state of Oregon decided by a 32,000 majority in favour of a 'Death With Dignity Act', Measure No. 16, which removed criminal penalties from doctors who prescribe drugs for patients to take their own lives. This law carries certain safeguards; it applies only to residents over eighteen years old, to qualify for a lethal prescription requires that one is suffering from a terminal disease which is defined as 'incurable and irreversible', and that the patient's decision is informed and voluntary. This latter safeguard would rule-out patients suffering from various depressive illnesses. Further safeguards include a requirement that the attending physician must provide information about the diagnosis, prognosis and risks associated with the prescribed medication and further information about 'feasible alternatives', and the opportunity to rescind the request. Notwithstanding this battery of safeguards, the state of Oregon have adopted a euthanasia policy and leaders of the euthanasia movement have already proclaimed it as a step towards active euthanasia. One of Oregon's critics, Alexander Morgan Capron, (1995) has demonstrated just how easy it can be to sidestep the alleged safeguards and make it possible to expand the programme in directions which are currently regarded as morally impermissible. Although less extreme than the failed initiatives in Washington and California the Oregon initiative, which allows a request for medication to terminate one's life, falls clearly within the category of euthanasia. The right to refuse therapy is morally and legally distinct from these initiatives; it cannot be interpreted as a right to die by lethal injection or administration of poison. The right to bodily integrity is the right to resist invasion; it does not involve the right to introduce whatever substances a person wishes. Hence laws protect against physical assault but prohibit the use of narcotics.

Advance directives are justified with reference to the 'right to refuse', and public and legal opinion increasingly recognises that an autonomous refusal should be upheld even if it results in death. Does this mean that an autonomous request for life-prolonging treatment should be given equal weight and respected accordingly? Apparently not. Whilst the right to refuse is based on a patient's entitlement to be free from bodily interference, which could amount to battery, there is no corresponding right to insist upon and receive whatever treatment one may desire. There is an analogy here with sexual activity. The right to refuse sexual activity is an acceptable exercise of autonomy, but there is no corresponding right to be provided with partners for sexual activity. However, the expectation that one should have a right to life-prolonging therapy should not be wholly undermined by such arguments. In a caring society people should expect that efforts would be made to prolong their lives if they so desire it, and those responsible for the allocation of health-care resources should expect severe criticism whenever lack of resources is responsible for an unwilling death.

Social Prejudice, Euthanasia and Advance Directives

There is, however, a common form of prejudice shared by many euthanasia and suicide rights activists as well as proponents of advance directives for discontinuation of therapy and medical cost-containment. Paul K. Longmore, (1987) a prominent disability rights activist, suggests that behind the so-called compassion of the arguments of 'suicide rights' activists is a form of hidden contempt for the disabled cloaking itself in paternalism. Longmore (1987:141) maintains that: 'explicitly or implicitly underlying their arguments, and the arguments of many medical cost-containment advocates as well, is a generally unquestioning adoption and reinforcement of social prejudices against people with disabilities, the elderly and even sick people.'

Citing dramatised pleas for assisted suicide and therapy withdrawal in popular films, such as *Whose Life is it Anyway?*, Longmore argues that these dramas reinforce the prejudice that disability robs people of their humanity, and encourage beliefs that the disabled are a burden on their families and society and that prolonging their existence denies resources to other disadvantaged minorities. These stories offer little indication of the possibilities for people with major disabilities to nevertheless work productively and have fulfilling relationships. They stress, instead, separation from the community and worthlessness, with death as the only choice in which an autonomous person can find release from misery.

A similar challenge to the negative stereotyping of disability can be seen in the arguments advanced by the English disability rights activist, Jenny Morris, (1993:59) who points out that disability is not '*in itself* sufficient to explain the intolerable nature of the life experienced.' She confronts the liberal humanist proponent of euthanasia:

> A liberal humanist approach to euthanasia may insist that individuals should be able to choose the manner and time of their death; that if somebody genuinely feels that their life is not worth living then they should not be forced to endure pain and suffering and unhappiness. But individuals do not exist within a vacuum.

> ...s of the society in which we
> live... ...hysical ability and perfection;
> ...those who do not conform to
> ...against disabled people do not
> just exist... ...they also reside within our
> own heads, particularly for those of us who become disabled in
> adult life. (Morris, 1993:44)

Morris also challenges the assumption - so frequently built into advance directives and pleas for physician-assisted suicide - that being disabled means that life is not worth living:

> The suicide of a disabled person is often treated as rational behaviour. No mental disturbance or emotional trauma is deemed necessary to explain the rejection of life by a disabled person. Instead their physical disability is taken as sufficient grounds to want to die. (Morris, 1993:44)

In recent evidence to the House of Lords Select Committee on Medical Ethics (1994:36) a spokesperson from ENABLE, an organisation concerned with the welfare of people with learning difficulties, endorsed Morris' point, stating that 'the actual quality of a disabled person's life often depends less on their disability, than on the way society treats the person.'

It is noteworthy that in the terminology of many advance directives the expressions 'terminally ill' and 'disabled' are ran together, thus reinforcing the prejudice that a disabled life is not worth extending. Morris and other disability rights activists reject this, maintaining that what makes life intolerable is not the disabled legs, but the steps, and asks whether the wish to die is not so much a rational response to disability but 'a desperate response to isolated oppression?' (Morris, 1993:42) Given the background conditions of economic deprivation and enforced social powerlessness then, as Longmore (1987:168) says: 'arguments for euthanasia, aid-in-dying, assisted suicide, and medical cost-containment simply rationalise the ultimate act of oppression,' and that 'advocates of assisted suicide assume a non-existent autonomy.'

One thing is clear: for disability rights activists such as Morris and Longmore, those who wish to extend control of treatment options to the point of assisted suicide are scarcely representative of the interests of the disabled. Says Longmore: (1987:167)

Reading through the literature of the suicide rights activists, one is struck by their willing acceptance of prejudicial assumptions about people with disabilities. Disability renders its 'victims' helpless and dependent. It robs them of the possibility of living meaningfully. It makes them emotionally, physically, and financially burdensome to themselves, their families, and society. One wades through reams of this suicide rights advocacy without finding any real acknowledgement of the intense social stigma and discrimination that segregate people with disabilities more than any contemporary minority, deny them opportunities for education, employment, marriage, and family, rob them of social dignity and esteem, and inflict on many of them what can only be called 'social death.'

It must be stressed that 'social death' is not a direct product of disability; it is a product of discrimination against disability.

Part of the appeal in advance directives is their tendency to run together arguments for autonomy with the desire to avoid an undignified dying process. To be sure, a life with little opportunity to exercise autonomy is bound up with our understanding of loss of dignity, but what is it that makes the illness undignified? Is it the pain, discomfort and disability? Or is it a combination of these together with societal prejudice against the perceived helplessness of frailty and disability? Cantor, (1993:55) who recognises that a living will should be relative to a person's concept of dignity, suggests that there are many factors which make life undignified:

> Physical pain, emotional suffering (feelings of embarrassment, frustration, and dependency), immobility and physical restraints, and physical appearance are common elements in defining an undignified or degrading state. Beyond personal well-being and dignity, a person might wish to consider the interests of surrounding persons - for example, loved ones and health-care providers. The interests of surrounding persons might include the emotional strain of protracted care, the economic costs of care, and the allocation of medical resources.

For Cantor the economic burdens of protracted health-care also provide an incentive for the withdrawal of therapy: 'Beyond the anguishing mental and physical burdens imposed upon surrounding persons, the economic cost of terminal care may be relevant.' (Cantor, 1993:65)

There is an unquestionable need for greater individual control when facing the above-mentioned aspects of an undignified life, but a document indicating therapy withdrawal and an early death is merely one of many options open to society. Better standards of health-care, counselling to combat emotional suffering and counselling and supportive assistance for relatives who may suffer emotional strain, are just some of the options available. In passages like these it is clear that prejudice against dependency is largely responsible for loss of dignity. Autonomy, on these terms, is equated with an abstract notion of individualism whereby it is degrading to be dependent upon other human beings. Death is thus presented as being preferable to dependency.

Proponents of living wills are not strictly concerned with the curtailment of an undignified dying process; the living will can be employed as an instrument to cut short an undignified existence where the condition is not life-threatening or terminal. As Cantor (1993:60) indicates:

> It is not unusual, for example, to see a living will which renounces life-sustaining medical intervention if the patient becomes permanently dependent on nursing care. That degree of helplessness and dependence, together with mental incompetence, represents an intolerably degrading spectre for these declarants.

Now Cantor acknowledges that living wills may be drawn up relative to a person's subjective concept of dignity. The problem is that our notions of dignity are not clearly subjective and personal; they are bound up with social beliefs and prejudices. Thus prejudices against incontinence, a wide range of disabilities, reliance upon others, and mental incapacity are already well-established as norms which are difficult to counter. A personal preference against continuing life with disability is merely a reinforcement of a dominant and even fashionable prejudice.

Whereas one of the original motives for advance directives lay in the attempt to maintain patient autonomy in a post-competent terminal state, current advocates of advance directives include references to the withholding of therapy that would leave the patient in a 'gravely debilitated state.' Thus Cantor (1993:15) observes: 'Often the patient's motive in rejecting medical intervention was distaste for the prospect of a gravely debilitated existence. (Among others, we are talking about the cancer patient, the gangrene patient, or the quadriplegic dependent on artificial aids).' The problem with this development is that when formalised in an advance directive, the expression 'gravely debilitated' is seen in a fixed sense related strictly to the patient's physical or mental disability, whereas being debilitated is bound up with many deprivations which could be avoided by the removal of social prejudice.

Conclusion

Advance directives have been promoted as a means of extending patient autonomy, but there are signs that they have not been so readily accepted as their original proponents predicted. The practical problems with them are not easily resolved with further intervention which, in any case, would involve a massive redirection of resources for counselling and assistance in their completion, educating surrogates, and arranging for reconsideration of the documents. Advance health-care documents have an appeal only to a minority of the population. Perhaps this could be recognised and it may be prudent to conclude that advance directives may be of great advantage to a minority who have the time, education, and sufficient access to medical counselling. For the bulk of the population they are unlikely to solve the problems they have promised to solve, and, if autonomy is their rationale, should only be encouraged from those who express a desire for them, have strong feelings or specific and unusual preferences - such as a wish not to be treated in a particular hospital again or an aversion to a particular therapy - rather than an ideal for which all should be encouraged to strive.

Turning to the problems of potential abuse of advance directives it is worth noting that at present pressure groups in favour of extending the scope of advance directives embrace both those who favour greater patient autonomy over therapy options and those who have an interest in killing. This is further complicated by the fact that the same movement can contain those whose interest in killing arises from compassion and those whose interest is grounded in fiscal or eugenic reasons.

Can proposals for autonomous treatment abatement be kept distinct from proposals for the right to kill? An affirmative answer would depend on NDA's and legislation concerning advance directives being framed in such a way that they do not support the long-term objectives of euthanasia societies; that 'aid-in-dying' amendments are recognized as proposals for the right to kill and consequently rejected. It is also necessary to state clearly and unambiguously that an autonomous refusal of certain forms of therapy - even if such refusal presents a life-threatening situation - is not equivalent to passive euthanasia. Thus legal directives which empower forms of therapy abatement should carry statements declaring opposition to euthanasia. The appeal to situations where one is 'better off dead' should be rejected as meaningless nonsense. Whatever ones views are concerning the worth of a particular life the option of being better off without it is vacuous. Being 'better off' implies some state of continued existence. It should be stressed that euthanasia is not really a relevant option for terminally ill patients either by act or omission. The main reason cited for a euthanasia request is intolerable pain and distress. It is far better to develop educational directions in pharmacological and other methods of reducing pain and distress and managing the terminally ill than repealing existing prohibitions on euthanasia and thus risking an undermining of the respect for life which is enshrined in good medical practice. It is certainly not the business of doctors, or ethicists, to accept the idea that some lives are not worth living. When therapy refusal is indicated the possibility of alternative therapy - rather than euthanasia - should be the medical profession's response.

IV 'Do Not Attempt to Resuscitate' Orders

Introduction

A particularly controversial aspect of therapy abatement in recent years has centred upon the ethical status of 'Do not attempt to resuscitate orders' (DNARs). The key ethical problems which are raised in relation to criteria for non-resuscitation can be expressed as follows: 1) Is there, or should there be, a limit to our obligation to save and prolong life? Related to this question is a much broader one: 2) When do moral values supersede objective medical wisdom? This chapter surveys the ethical issues surrounding DNAR orders, considers objections to them, and proposes guidelines for issuing DNAR orders which are based jointly on self-determination and limited paternalism.

DNAR and CPR

Cardiac arrest occurs at some point in the dying process of every person whatever the underlying cause of death. In this respect CPR (cardio-pulmonary resuscitation) is potentially relevant for all terminally ill hospital patients. DNAR orders are generally understood as requirements to withhold CPR in certain cases, although the exact meaning of CPR is not always clear. CPR involves external chest compression and some forms of artificial respiration. Resuscitation after cardiac arrest involves a series of steps towards sustaining adequate circulation of blood to vital organs whilst heartbeat is restored. CPR was introduced in the 1960s, but did not achieve full approval of the American Heart Associated until 1974. (Youngner, 1987:24) In 1960 W.B. Kouwenhoven *et al* published their results of impressive recoveries after cardiac arrest with a new technique of closed-chest cardiac massage coupled with, if required, a defibrillator. This required no special surgical skills and could be carried out by a doctor or paramedic or even a lay person with adequate training. Throughout the 1960's major hospitals in the USA and Europe set up emergency teams to employ resuscitative skills at the bedside of anyone suffering from cardiac arrest in hospital. Before application of modern techniques of CPR, death was an inevitable outcome of cessation of heartbeat and respiration. Although initially designed for healthy persons who suffered cardiac arrest during surgery, or near drowning accident victims, resuscitation procedures are now used on numerous patients, of varying states of health, who suffer cardiac arrest in hospital. No doubt many lives have been saved by CPR but it has raised problems. In principle it is possible for almost any dying patient to be resuscitated and survive for a short while. It has been argued that instead of a peaceful death some patients near the end of life could be victims of the technological imperative, undergoing futile but aggressive attempts at life-prolongation. Given the framework for ethical decision-making - established in Chapter II - which involved a transition from duties to the living and duties to the dying, it is important to consider when CPR is part of the medical staff's duty. It is clearly necessary to consider policies for deciding between those for whom resuscitation attempts are relevant and those for whom they are not. But who is to decide? A purely medical decision suggests paternalism, which many find objectionable in an era where patient autonomy is exalted. Nevertheless, some form of limited paternalism will be defended here, and it will be maintained that it is not incompatible with the principle of respect for patient autonomy.

Not every attempt at CPR is successful and in the majority of cases it probably fails to sustain life. According to Dan English (1994:94) CPR has a mixed success employed on around one-third dying patients in US hospitals. Of these one-third survive after CPR and one-third of *those* survive until hospital discharge. English notes, in this context, the semantic fallacy in the expression DNR, which implies that resuscitation can be achieved. He correctly prefers the expression DNAR (Do Not Attempt to Resuscitate) as a more realistic terminology would enhance realistic decision-making. CPR is an effective and beneficial form of therapy for a small number of patients; for many it is a desperate measure with little prospect of success. (Saunders 1994:86)

Criteria for Issuing DNAR Orders

After cardiac arrest delay in administering CPR reduces the efficiency of the effort to resuscitate. Hence decisions on whether or not to perform CPR are best settled in advance. Do not attempt to resuscitate orders, and the debate regarding their ethical status, have emerged in the context of providing criteria for the withholding or application of CPR. In the opinion of many professional organizations in health-care DNAR orders are appropriate when it is agreed that a patient's well-being will not be served by CPR. For example, CPR is not indicated in certain situations involving advanced terminal illness.

The two main reasons given for issuing a DNAR order are 1] if the patient has indicated a previous autonomous refusal, and 2] if resuscitation is deemed 'medically inappropriate' or 'futile' by the doctors. According to the Judicial Affairs Committee of the American Medical Association (AMA, 1991) some 88% of DNAR orders in US hospitals are based in part on the doctor's judgement that CPR would be futile. (The concepts of 'medically inappropriate' and 'futility' are bound up with further complex moral issues and will be addressed in the following chapter.) As cardiac and respiratory failure is an inevitable part of the dying process, there is no reason why CPR could not be employed on every patient prior to death. John Saunders (1994) considers the ethics of universal CPR. The argument that it would maximise the number of lives saved whilst doing no harm, as the terminally ill would surely die with or without it, is rejected. Saunders points out that CPR can be harmful; it can harm the patient whose remaining hours of life are spent enduring physical assault; it is distressing to other patients, relations who have to cope with thwarted attempts at resuscitation, and the health-care staff whose morale is lowered by unsuccessful attempts to resuscitate hopeless cases. This can, as Saunders points out, lead to cynicism among health-care workers. Quite obviously it is morally offensive to perform full-scale resuscitation on every dying patient, but an area of ethical concern lies in certain borderline cases involving the application of CPR to certain categories of terminally or critically ill patients.

CPR is a very dramatic intervention, and this aspect highlights certain ethical issues. In a hospital, cardiac or respiratory arrest normally initiates a swirl of activity, with doctors, nurses and technicians, racing to the bed in an apparent attempt to 'bring a patient back from the dead' or at least 'to snatch someone from the jaws of death'. This dramatic element is deeply ingrained in the public perception of medicine. In every television hospital soap series CPR dramatically presents doctors and nurses as champions in a war with death itself. Unlike other organ failures, where there might be time for reflection, cardiac arrest requires instant attention. In contrast, a decision not to resuscitate involves no dramatic display of action; relatives and nurses simply wait at the bedside until the doctor pronounces the patient dead. It is partly the dramatic nature of CPR intervention which explains why many physicians find it difficult to accept a DNAR in the same way as they might accept the withholding of chemotherapy or palliative surgery. The same might be said of relatives who find a DNAR decision disturbing. When confronting sudden death we are frequently accustomed to valiant efforts, risk taking, no expense spared, to save a life. The passive acceptance of someone's death does not come easily for most people.

Moreover, withholding CPR is not like withholding certain forms of surgical intervention, where one can weigh up the relative risks and alternatives. There is no middle course where a patient can be made comfortable, be given alternative therapy and an opportunity to prepare for possible death - as opposed to risking death during surgery. With CPR there is only emergency. As Kathleen Nolan (1987:12) says: 'if surgery is withheld there is always a risk of death, while if resuscitation is withheld there is a certainty of death'.

There is considerable resistance to the refusal of CPR in the operating theatre. It would seem that physicians who are willing to comply with a DNAR order, when CPR would prolong the agony of a dying patient, have reservations when such a patient has a cardiac arrest in the operating theatre. This may stem from the belief that it is morally acceptable to withhold CPR after 'natural' arrest, but that it is morally questionable to withhold it after physician - i.e. anaesthesia - induced arrest. A test case might be the following. A patient in prior consultation with the doctors decides not to have CPR in the event of an arrest but is willing to accept other forms of therapy including surgery. The patient is later admitted for minor surgery and suffers a cardiac arrest in the operating theatre. In such cases there is a reluctance to withhold resuscitation. It might be argued that the arrest is physician induced and that doctors would be reluctant to accept a DNAR order in such circumstances. A partial solution to this problem would be to clarify instructions regarding CPR, such that the DNAR order states that either operating theatre arrests are included or not. In general, however, a limited form of paternalism should prevail in relation to patients admitted for surgical intervention, as enforcement of DNAR orders in such settings may conflict with the moral *raison d'etre* of surgical procedures.

It should be noted that in the perioperative setting most of the measures employed for resuscitation are already in routine use. In the event of an arrest the only additional intervention is the employment of CPR. Moreover, DNAR orders are bound up with policies whereby patients are allowed to die, whereas the whole ethos of the operating theatre is towards efforts at life-prolongation. This is because perioperative treatment is life-threatening and invasive, where patients are put at risk for a short period with the overall objective that the patient will emerge alive and in some way better off than before the operation. The justification of the risks of anaesthesia and surgery is that it is known that every effort must be made to help patients survive it. Its very point would be compromised if guidelines were introduced to facilitate an early death in the operating theatre. It is expected of surgeons to recommend patients against any form of surgical intervention whose outcome is potentially lethal. Thus, according to Cynthia B. Cohen and Peter J. Cohen:(1992:358) 'To retain DNAR orders in the perioperative setting and allow patients to die of reversible arrest conflicts with the very goals for which patients undergo surgery'. This would indicate a strong case for advising patients and relatives to suspend DNAR requests during the perioperative phase as it involves interventions which are a matter of routine in the operating theatre. A similar case might be made in favour of waiving DNAR orders for patients undergoing electro-convulsion therapy.

The Intensive Care Unit (ICU) is problematic for DNAR orders. In fact a patient for whom no CPR is indicated would not benefit from intensive care. The ICU differs from other medical settings in a number of important respects. In his study of ICU medicine, Robert Zussman (1992:36) points out that 'Intensive care... is organised around a notion that medicine at its best - at its most heroic, its purest - is about physiology and physiology alone.' He cites a resident's description of the ICU's mission: 'The unit... is really a place to get people over a kind of medical disaster. Its a place you just try to get them out of alive, and you don't worry about (other things). You treat the immediate problem.' (*ibid*:37) In other settings medicine's critics complain that the patient is reduced to a disease; in an ICU even the disease may take a secondary role. Says Zussman: 'in intensive care physicians may focus on a particular physiological process in which even the underlying disease is forgotten.' (*ibid*:37) The ICU is not an environment for the consideration of advance directives or patient's preferences regarding CPR. Such decisions should be taken before admission, or if taken later they should focus on removal from the unit.

Resistance to issuing DNAR orders may be attributed in part to the connection between resuscitation and the traditional cardio-respiratory concept of death. Resuscitation has frequently been spoken of as a reversal of death, bringing back life to the pulseless and non-breathing patient. Nowadays brain-related criteria for death has focused attention on the very meaning of CPR which, prior to brainstem definitions of death, was seen as a means of bringing back to life those who were 'clinically dead'. Thus CPR has metaphorically, and in some cases literally, been equated with resurrection, giving doctors god-like powers over life and death. Historically, loss of heart-beat and respiration was an irreversible condition, but success in resuscitation since the late 1950s contributed to a change in this perception. Successful heart-lung transplants, together with recognition that loss of brainstem function is the ultimate mechanism of death, have reconstituted the very meaning of death. We now have a situation where prolonged cardio-respiratory function is independent of the boundary between life and death. Quite clearly no doctor has an ethical obligation to indefinitely maintain the semblance of life in a brain dead heart-lung preparation, other than in those instances where transplant organs are required. (Lamb, 1985)

Guidelines for issuing DNAR orders could be derived possibly from the distinction between 1) CPR as a means of 'curative restoration' and 2) CPR as a means of 'life prolongation'. Curative restoration would include those cases where CPR is bound up with a strategy aimed at complete restoration, as in cases of drowning or electrocution. In another context resuscitation might be performed in order to sustain life during a period of initial diagnosis of therapy, as in cases involving drug overdose. In these cases the passive withholding of resuscitative support would be hard to distinguish from euthanasia, or at least professional misconduct.

In many contexts resuscitation may be less curative than life-prolonging. It is here that serious ethical assessment is necessary, especially in cases where death is delayed without hope of cure, improvement of help or relief of suffering, merely to prolong biological function with no possible benefit to the patient. A point may be reached where CPR falls into a category of hopeless or *futile* therapy. This might then provide an ethical justification for a DNAR order. For under such conditions CPR can be of no benefit and extremely distressing, as can be illustrated by the following example:

> Mrs. R was a thirty five year old woman who had developed progressive liver failure and an accumulation of fluid in the

peritoneal cavity following ilial bypass one year earlier for the treatment of obesity; at the time of surgery she weighed 260 pounds. She had also developed a severe gastrointestinal bleed, inflammation of the brain, and kidney failure. At MICU admission, Mrs. R weighed 100 pounds. Her swollen abdomen contrasted grossly with her emaciated frame and elf-like face. She was being treated with blood transfusions, intravenous feeding, haemodialysis, vasopressors, and repeated tappings to remove the fluid accumulating in the abdominal and chest cavities. The intern was afraid of a full resuscitation attempt in the event of cardiac arrest. 'When we grab hold of her to turn her', he said, 'the skin comes off in big pieces down to the mid-dermis. When you move her you can feel her tiny brittle ribs moving in and out of their joints. My God! If we perform CPR on this poor women we literally break her into pieces. (cited by Youngner, 1987:24)

Cases like this test the ethical limits of CPR and indicate a need for further assessment of DNAR guidelines. In keeping with the principles of beneficence and respect for patient autonomy any modification to the guidelines should be primarily in the patient's interest.

The President's Commission (1983) outlined three ethical principles in the context of DNAR orders. They are self-determination, well-being and equity. Respect for the principle of self-determination involves a recognition that different patients will have different needs and concerns at the ends of their lives, and will place different values on the prospect of more or less time available to them. There are, however, major problems in meeting criteria for a self-determined decision not to accept CPR, as crucial to the decision-making process is the initiation of a discussion about a DNAR order and its consequences. For example, it would be downright cruel to initiate a discussion on the prospect of foregoing CPR with some patients whilst others may be capable of handling it without undue distress. Respect for the patient's well-being may clash with a duty to respect self-determination. Now judgements about a patient's well-being are based on assessments of the alleged benefits of a particular therapy. There may be considerable disparity between the patient's and the doctor's concept of well-being and the patient may not fully understand the consequences of a therapeutic decision or have adequate knowledge of alternatives and their consequences.

The principle of equity has given rise to a number of ethical dilemmas in intensive care. Some have argued that in the interests of equity CPR should be withheld from certain patients who cannot benefit - such as those suffering from a major organ failure -if its cost, together with the backup treatment, denies treatment to others who could benefit from access to medical resources. Proposals to withhold CPR for cost-containment reasons could introduce situations where medical personnel appeared callous, making cold calculations, resisting pleas for continuation of therapy. There is no doubt, that in a world where resources are scarce, such calculations unfortunately take place. But they should not be wholly endorsed by ethical principles; rather it should be argued on moral grounds that CPR should be provided, that patients should have access to it, if they need it and if they have not indicated a preference to the contrary. Resuscitation, when applied in the patient's best interests, provides benefits that justify the costs. It may be that non-resuscitation of certain individuals may benefit society in that it releases resources for other patients, but that should never be the reason for it.

Among the problems in ascertaining a valid form of patient consent to a DNAR order are the following: a patient who constantly changes his mind from day to day; a wish not to be a nuisance to others, depression, and fears to express views which conflict with those known to be held by relatives.

Cynthia Cohen and Peter Cohen (1992) review six categories where DNAR orders may be morally justified: 1) patients who will die imminently; 2) patients with irreversible illness such as advanced cancer and limited life expectancy. Whilst resuscitation would postpone death it would offer no benefit to outweigh the burden of continuous treatments. 3) Patients in whom arrest would signal deterioration, leading either to death or severe deficits unacceptable to them. For example, patients with reason to fear that resuscitation would place them at risk of permanent brain injury or substantial morbidity. 4) Patients for whom resuscitation would be physiologically futile, where futility means that there is no reasonable probability that it would re-establish heartbeat and prevent death. 5) Patients for whom resuscitation would offer only a small probability of survival; for example, metastatic cancer, sepsis, acute stroke, or pneumonia approaching zero. 6) Finally, where resuscitation would be both invasive and painful. For example, patients with chronic conditions, such as osteoporosis, where illness precluded survival of the rigours of CPR. Cohen and Cohen suggest that surgery may also be limited in some of these categories, although it may be warranted in categories 2, 3, 5 and 6, but not for 1, and very unlikely for 4. Patients in category 5 might be offered surgery, as the success rate of resuscitation during anaesthesia and surgery is comparatively high and palliation in the post-operative stage would make it possible for patients in category 6. DNAR decisions could be based on computer analysis of APACHE (Acute Physiology and Chronic Health Evaluation) scores, although it is generally agreed that such data should not be used rigorously as patient non-survival of CPR is not wholly predictable.

In some cases, because of the violence, the isolation, and mere prolongation of life with no possibility of benefits, many patients might have a genuine interest in not being resuscitated. This need not be interpreted as a suicidal intention - even when death is the inevitable outcome - nor should compliance with such a wish be seen as a form of passive euthanasia. It may be nothing more than an aversion to certain forms of therapy. If such a desire were strongly presented one could appreciate a management strategy which excluded resuscitation, provided that this preference had been clearly indicated by the patient. Many published guidelines stress that 'No CPR' does not mean 'no therapy' or 'no caring'. Other forms of support may be carried out, including opening and cleaning airways, providing oxygen per nasal cannula, and efforts to make the patient comfortable together with the provision of emotional support to the patient and members of the family. Surgery may be performed on a patient with a DNAR order, and the same moral requirements would apply in this case as with other patients; namely that surgery must offer the prospect of some benefit, cure, amelioration, maintenance or palliation. For example, a patient may have a DNAR order only in relation to cardiac disease, but benefit from surgical treatment relating to a kidney stone. A patient who can no longer ingest food orally may benefit from the surgical insertion of a feeding tube. (Cohen and Cohen, 1992)

Not all DNAR decisions are bound up with hospital management strategies. The following scenario is indicative of problems bound up with the implementation of advance directives to withhold CPR outside of the hospital. A terminally ill cancer patient being cared for at home begins vomiting blood and goes into cardiac arrest. An ambulance is called and the emergency medical team, under a legal and professional imperative to resuscitate, initiate CPR despite the family's protests, resulting in verbal and physical abuse. This example clearly indicates a need for further discussion on guidelines for DNAR orders outside of hospital, especially with terminal patients with cancer or AIDS who have elected for home or hospice care. Emergency ambulance teams are required to initiate resuscitation which, in some cases, may frustrate the wishes of the patient. One suggestion is that patients not wishing to be resuscitated should wear a bracelet with a DNAR request on it. Thus facilities have evolved in the US where, for example, terminal cancer patients or AIDS patients may wear an EMS (Emergency Medical Service) bracelet which specifies the withholding of CPR. Patient bracelets, worn by patients outside of hospital, who have signed an advance directive indicating a preference for certain therapeutic measures to be withheld, have been accepted in many US states.

It should be stressed, however, that the significance of an informed decision not to resuscitate is bound up with a shift from seeing CPR as a curative intervention to seeing it as a life-prolonging one.

The following guidelines for DNAR orders could be formulated:

1) *DNAR orders should specify exactly which treatment options should be withheld* These should not be couched in vague or imprecise terms like 'extraordinary', 'heroic', or 'aggressive therapy', which may have a variety of meanings to different individuals. A DNAR order is meaningless unless one understands the rationale behind it. Simply issuing a DNAR order without precise guidelines - for example, without an explicit reference to CPR - might be interpreted as an order for passive euthanasia. DNAR orders should be solely in respect to CPR. But there is also a need to be specific with regard to CPR, which itself covers a range of activities from chest-thumping, bone-crunching, electric shocks, to less invasive measures, such as drug support and fluid resuscitation.

A DNAR order should therefore specify which type of CPR should be withheld. If the exclusion of CPR is part of a management strategy then euthanasia will not be an issue. It should also be stressed that a DNAR order which specifies the withholding of CPR is not a decision to abandon to let die but, in certain cases, indicates a refusal to continue with one form of futile therapy. It is not a decision to kill, and when appropriate, other therapy, such as transfusions and antibiotics, should not be influenced by a DNAR order.

2) *Patients and families, and nursing staff should participate wherever possible in DNAR decisions* There is a need for discussion between doctors and patients on whether or not to initiate CPR in eventual cardiac

arrest. Discussions might therefore be initiated with patients who are at risk from cardiac failure or arrest. This is not an easy matter. There are degrees of comprehension, and there are often reduced levels of consciousness when decisions are near. Hard pressed doctors do not always have time to discuss options fully, and decision- making in this context requires a sense of urgency. There are problems interpreting a family request to 'do everything possible'. Is this a judgement in the patients best interest or an expression of guilt? What if the family's perceptions are distorted by false hopes? In these circumstances can we say that the doctor knows best? In any doubtful circumstances a presumption in favour of life should be operative, and no doctor should ever be censured for acting in accord with it. This view was endorsed by the President's Commission, (1983:240) which supported a 'presumption in favour of resuscitation' when no clear advance deliberation had been indicated. The contribution of nurses in DNAR decision-making is significant and their close contact with patients and relatives indicates the importance of this role.

Of course it is advantageous if therapeutic decision-making is taken at a time when the patient is most competent. But how is a competent decision to be determined? Should all patients be asked about DNAR options on entering a hospital? It is difficult to discuss DNAR decisions with patients and in practice in the UK such discussion is the exception rather than the rule. (Saunders, 1994:79) The problem here is that one does not wish to upset patients at a time when their condition is not serious, but later, when they are less competent, it may be too late for an informed decision. Not all of the difficulties in implementing DNAR orders can be resolved by advanced directives, and prior consent may, in certain cases, have to be overruled by the moral principles and practical wisdom of the physician.

Saunders offers two compelling cases in support for a doctrine of limited paternalism regarding DNAR orders.

1. A slightly deaf, wheezy, bronchitic, elderly patient presents with central severe chest pain in an emergency department. Does he at 85 really want CPR? How do we inform him of the possible need for CPR, the technique and its outcome, the experience of intensive care, of ventilators and mental impairment and institutionalisation and all the rest, and then assure ourselves that his understanding is not impaired by senile dementia and his consent is informed, that he is truly

competent? (Saunders, 1994:79-80)

2. Consider a bride and groom involved in a major accident on their wedding night. One is killed, the other seriously injured. Although the survivor passes all the conventional tests of mental competence, would a request for a DNAR order be implemented by a good doctor? Surely it would be overruled and justifiably so, on the grounds that it represents an impulsive opinion, that would never be taken apart from short-lived special circumstances. (*ibid*:80-81)

Conclusion

Uncertainty in drawing the line between patient autonomy and deference to medical wisdom is partly bound up with the fact that attitudes are in a transitional stage. Although there is an attitudinal shift in favour of patient autonomy and informed consent, we are still very far from a situation where it is desirable for patient autonomy to completely override appeals to medical wisdom. In some contexts, such as the operating theatre or the ICU, and when there is uncertainty regarding the patient's wishes, the principle of limited paternalism should be uppermost and a presumption in favour of life should outweigh other considerations. Although it is important to ascertain a patient's known preferences a DNAR decision requires more discussion than any other option to forego therapy. This emphasises that it should not be a momentary decision which can be rescinded. Guidelines on DNAR orders should consequently reflect this important discursive element.

V Futile Therapy

Introduction

This chapter will investigate the notion of futile therapy and the ethical dilemmas which have emerged in recent discussions concerning criteria for the withholding of therapy which is regarded as 'futile' or 'medically inappropriate'. Insistence on the right to refuse to administer futile therapy could be described as a form of physician autonomy which imposes limits on patient autonomy. Of course patient autonomy is not the most fundamental principle in medical ethics. It is scarcely invoked in support of a patient who wants to be kept permanently in a persistent vegetative state or a demand for a therapy which a doctor knows to be unprofessional or a demand to be given preferential treatment over others. The issue to be decided, however, is the ethical basis of physician autonomy - the right to determine what therapy is medically appropriate or futile. It will be argued here that the determination of futile therapy is primarily a moral issue rather than a factual scientific one, but that doctors and health-care providers as moral agents have a duty to recognise and implement such criteria. In this respect the determination of futile therapy conforms to the principle of limited paternalism, which recognises that doctors have a moral obligation to act in their patients' best interests whilst recognising valid claims for a patient's self-determination. This, of course, requires a discussion of where to draw the line in particular cases and a full analysis of the concept of futile therapy.

Medical Futility

Whilst doctors have an ethical responsibility to respect an autonomous patient's wish for life-prolonging treatment there is a consensus amongst professionals that this imperative must be bounded by the application of criteria for futile therapy. The question that will be addressed here is when are physicians ethically permitted to refrain from providing what they regard as futile medical intervention?

This problem has been exacerbated in cases involving incompetent patients where surrogates have been accused of either frustrating a patient's wish or frustrating the doctor's practice of good medicine. In recent years open conflicts have become more prevalent between doctors and patients or surrogates who have sought treatment that their doctors have regarded as medically inappropriate, and there is a 'growing number of physicians and health-care institutions [who] exhibit a willingness to challenge such demands'. (Kapp, 1994:170) In Mrs. R's case, which was discussed in the previous chapter, CPR was deemed to be futile because the attempt would literally break her into pieces, and it is generally agreed that it is irrational to provide CPR when it would be futile. But there has been little discussion of the concept and criteria for futility, and philosophers have until fairly recently assumed that discussion about futile therapy falls wholly within the sphere of medical expertise. This is not strictly correct and betrays a residual commitment to a positivist distinction between inquiries into factual matters and values. The problem of defining medical futility has become acute in the light of a growing number of court rulings which have turned on appeals to therapy which is considered 'medically inappropriate'. In 1991 Daniel Callaghan of the Hastings Center described the problem of defining futility as 'the problem without a name'. He saw futility as the other side of 'medical necessity', which is also hard to define as we lack a coherent view of the ends of medicine. Giles Scofield (1991:31) has expressed doubts concerning the claim that medical expertise conveys some insight into the nature of futile therapy: 'The belief that physicians know futility when they see it is an illusion. There is no set definition of medical futility, only suggested parameters that vary widely.' The term 'futility' is derived from the Latin word *'futilis'*, which means 'leaky'. This in turn is derived from Greek mythology which records how the daughters of Daneus were sent to Hades where they were condemned to draw water in leaky vessels, which meant that they could never achieve the objective of their actions. But when we speak of medical futility the problem is compounded by the fact that there is very often uncertainty regarding the overall objectives. For example it is not always certain that a therapy is judged to be futile because it simply will not bring about any physiological improvement or arrest a deteriorating condition, or whether it is judged to be futile because in the eyes of the medical team it is unlikely to improve the patient's quality of life. Here one might consider whether it is futile to continue to provide life-sustaining therapy when the patient has no likelihood of regaining consciousness. If futile therapy is defined in terms of it not being likely to improve the quality of the patient's life it would seem to be futile to resuscitate PVS patients. This kind of judgement involves moral, political and economic issues as well as medical knowledge. In an essential sense the problem of futility is a moral one. It will be argued here that physicians are moral agents and should not be confined to the expression of opinions of matters of medical fact. A distinction between the concept and criteria for futility might be useful at this point. In a very important sense the definition of 'medical futility' is very much a matter for the philosopher or bioethicist, whilst the application for criteria would rest partly with the doctor and partly with an informed patient. This means that both doctor and patient are aware of the moral and philosophical aspects of futility, which includes assessment and evaluation of quality of life. A recognition of the moral dimensions of the debate on medical futility is bound up with the increasing value placed on respect for autonomy and informed consent which calls for a more interactive doctor-patient relationship.

Although there is no consensus at present over the definition, meaning and criteria for futility some progress has been made with the concept of physiological futility which refers to a treatment that is 'clearly futile in achieving its physiologic objective and so offers no benefit to the patient'. (Hastings Center Guidelines, 1987:32) A paradigm case would be a seventy-five-year-old patient with end-stage metastatic cancer. In the event of an arrest cardiac resuscitation would be deemed physiologically futile because there is no chance of achieving the physiological objective, namely restoration of a functioning cardiac rhythm. This would appear to be a morally commendable decision, although it might be conceded that a level of certainty cannot be absolutely guaranteed for all patients in that condition. For whilst it is clearly wrong to provide CPR when it is futile, as a general rule, it may be difficult to decide in particular cases whether CPR is actually futile. Nevertheless, the statute on CPR issued by the New York State (1987) would seem to be correct when it says that 'medically futile means that CPR will be unsuccessful in restoring cardiac and respiratory function or the patient will experience repeated arrests in a short time period before death occurs'. Implants of mechanical hearts or baboon-human heart transplants may also be regarded as futile forms of therapy but may be appropriate as a bridge which can maintain the patient until a suitable transplantable organ is found. Strictly speaking CPR is futile when it offers no benefit to the patient because maximal therapy has failed and no physiological improvement is possible. Under these circumstances a unilateral decision by physicians to withhold CPR would seem to be in order. But such judgements may encompass a wide range of probabilities and evaluations. Some doctors see CPR as futile if the probability of success is 0%, others rate it as high as 13% (AMA, 1992:1870) Further differences can be found in criteria employed to evaluate the outcome of CPR. It is indisputably futile if it fails to restore heartbeat, but is it futile if heartbeat is restored but the patient is left in a state of permanent unconsciousness? This latter case involves a moral judgement concerning the quality of such a life. Doctors also vary in the boundaries for survival after CPR. Some might see CPR as appropriate if it leads to survival for 24 hours or until the patient is released from hospital. Others employ a longer survival time-scale, such as one or even six months after the initial cardiac arrest. With this degree of flexibility in determining the appropriateness or futility of CPR there is opportunity for patients and their doctors to evaluate objectives in an ongoing dialogue.

The expressions 'medically inappropriate' or 'futile therapy' involve a range of judgements. They can refer to therapy which has been shown to have no use, such as laetrile's ineffectiveness as a cure for cancer, or Mrs. Jones' 'pick-me-up' which has no medical meaning beyond the relationship between a particular patient and her doctor, and cases where overwhelming medical trials have demonstrated that a certain course of therapy is unlikely to bring benefit and could even involve further risk. Here the facts, based on evidence and probability surveys, may be regarded as beyond dispute and consequently admit of no moral objections. But 'futile' can have another meaning which admits moral contestability, especially when therapy is deemed to be futile because it does not bring about any significant improvement in the quality of life.

The Appleton Conference (1992:6) acknowledged a distinction between two meanings of 'futility': the first involves 'physiologically' futile treatments, where the desired change cannot be achieved, and the second involves a low probability of success or a low quality of life that is likely after the proposed treatment. In the latter case they recommended that a decision to withhold therapy should only be made in the context of 'full and open discussion of the nature and extent of the "futility" of the treatment with the patient's representatives'.

Given the scope for disagreement whether the goal is futile or not it is important not to confuse 'futility' in the strong sense, which refers to a therapy that cannot bring about a desired physiological change, with 'futility' in the weak sense, which refers to a therapy that cannot bring improvement in quality of life. This latter case admits a wide range of value judgements with scope for challenges to the ethical values which may underpin a doctor's criterion of futility.

One example of the strong sense of 'futility' is to be found in an act on DNAR orders adopted by the State of Georgia, which defines medical futility as a resuscitative effort that 'will likely be unsuccessful in restoring cardiac and respiratory function or will only restore cardiac and respiratory function for a brief period of time so that the patient will likely experience need for cardiopulmonary resuscitation over a short period of time'. (cited by A.M. Capron, 1991:27) Of course the terms 'brief', 'short', and 'likely' need to be quantified, but as A.M. Capron (1991:28) points out this act avoids equating 'futility' with a 'condition of continued existence that does not seem worth sustaining in the eyes of the medical team'.

In an instructive footnote to the Appleton Conference (1992:8) Howard Brody drew attention to four categories of futility which have emerged in recent discussions on the ethical issues involved. First, where treatment is unlikely to achieve its physiological objective. Second, where the treatment may achieve its physiological objective but leave the patient in a state which is regarded as undesirable by the medical profession. This might involve a state of severe pain, gross mutilation, or loss of function. Third, the treatment may achieve its physiological objective but is likely to produce consequences deemed unacceptable by the vast majority of people. Fourth, the treatment may produce benefits in the patient's eyes, but in the doctor's opinion the treatment is futile because the perceived burdens far outweigh the benefits.

On reflection it appears that the first category is entirely non-controversial. In the fourth category, argues Brody, it would be wrong to withhold treatment and to use the word 'futility' in support of the decision. But categories two and three contain morally contestable situations which are bound up with perceptions regarding the kind of consequences which are regarded as unacceptable. Although Brody offers no examples to illustrate the problems with categories two and three it is not difficult to outline them. For example, the degree of suffering mentioned in category two may reflect a wide range of subjective beliefs and varying levels of pain thresholds. This has been observed in controversies bound up with decisions to withhold corrective surgery from infants suffering from Downs Syndrome or spina bifida on the grounds that it would be futile. In the case of Baby Jane Doe corrective surgery was withheld on the basis of predictions that she was doomed to spend the rest of her life bed-ridden and institutionalised. But in retrospect, argues Edward R. Grant, (1992:331) 'the surgery would have been effective in enhancing the quality of her life'. Disability activists have also argued that levels of suffering and disability may not in themselves warrant discontinuation of life-prolonging therapy. In category three, cultural beliefs may play an influential part when reflecting on the nature of unacceptable consequences. For example, cultural attitudes towards xenografts and hostility to the use of primates as organ sources, might be considered as part of the assessment of unacceptable consequences. More sinister, perhaps, is the possibility that medical futility may reinforce forms of discrimination already practised against the disabled, as seen in the evaluation of therapeutic intervention on infants with Downs' Syndrome and spina bifida.

In an interview in *The Guardian*, 26 October, 1986, a disabled person replied very firmly to the discriminatory aspects of futility judgements:

> Thank God this 'abnormal' foetus was conceived in 1947. I was born with spina bifida. My parents were told I would die within three days (wrong!), wouldn't walk (wrong!) and would be ineducable (wrong!)...
> Years ago we kept 'the handicapped' in institutions, out of sight, out of mind. Now (prenatal diagnosis and abortion), we can destroy them before we need to look at them or think of them. But we the handicapped are still *here*, still playing a part in society. Funnily enough, not only do many of us contribute to society, *we even enjoy being alive*.

Defensive and Offensive futility

In legal decisions in both the UK and the USA two forms of the appeal to futility have emerged. These have been described as defensive and offensive futility respectively. (Grant, 1992) Defensive futility is usually resorted to when the doctors and the family jointly agree that a particular form of life support should no longer be employed. This was seen in the court's decision in *Quinlan* and the House of Lords decision in *Airedale NHS Trust v Bland* (1993). The appeal to futility was employed as a defence against charges that withdrawal of life-sustaining therapy is a form of homicide or euthanasia, as the providers of therapy are not legally required to provide futile therapy.

The second concept of futility - offensive futility - is sometimes called 'physician autonomy' and is more recent. It has emerged in cases where health-care workers have challenged a patient or relative's request for a continuation of therapy. According to Grant offensive futility raises no new principles and analysis should therefore proceed from the same principle for both concepts of futility, and lead to similar outcomes. One might, however, object that 'offensive futility' may be perceived as an assault on the patient or the relative's autonomy, as in *Wanglie*. And Grant notes that a double standard is sometimes apparent. For example, the autonomous patient is said to know best as long as he/she exercises a right to an advance directive specifying a wish to forego certain forms of therapy, but if the patient insists on receiving therapy, then the doctor knows best.

The question of offensive futility emerged in the UK in March, 1995 and involved a decision to withhold further chemotherapy and a bone-marrow transplant from a ten-year-old girl suffering from leukaemia. In mid-January, 1995, her doctors had predicted that she only had six to eight weeks to live. In March, 1995, the Cambridge Health Authority refused to provide the therapy; they appealed to the futility of such treatment in her case, maintaining that she had less than a 3% chance of survival. They also appealed to 'tight resources' and made suggestions in the press that the £75,000 her treatment would cost could be better spent on other patients. Conducting their appeal on the grounds of offensive futility the health authority spent £15,000 on legal fees which, ironically, was what the chemotherapy would have cost. The girl's father appealed to the High Court and Mr. Justice Laws ruled that the health authority should reconsider its decision to withhold treatment. Within 24 hours, the Court of Appeal, led by Sir Thomas Bingham, ruled on 10 March, 1995 in favour of the health authority. His ruling indicated that offensive futility should be linked to the cost of therapy and he endorsed utilitarian criteria for health-care rationing when he said: 'Difficult and agonizing judgements have to be made as to how a limited budget is best allocated to the maximum advantage of the maximum number of patients'. (Reported in *The Independent*, 11 March, 1995:1)

Immediately after the Appeal Court's ruling, offers to provide funds were made and an anonymous donor eventually paid for the therapy which the girl received at a private clinic. On 3 May, 1995 a BBC radio news report indicated that the girl had responded to the treatment, was in remission and was looking forward to returning to school. But the case revealed how criteria for offensive futility and physician involvement with cost-containment policies are intertwined. Despite claims that the case brought implicit health-care rationing into the open, the courts had apparently endorsed a process of secret decision-making which takes place in NHS trusts, and has little scope for public involvement or respect for patient autonomy.

Hidden Values in Futility Judgements

Ronald Crawford and Lawrence Gostin (1992) suggest several ways in which the term 'futility' has been applied in value-laden ways. First, they note that treatment is regarded as futile if it will not improve the quality and duration of the patient's life and will not result in any improvement in the patient's physical or mental condition. For example, it is argued that continuous ventilatory support for long term PVS patients 'does not serve the goal of restoring them to any kind of cognitive life'. But whilst this fails to meet the medical goal of improving quality of life it is still a matter of moral concern as to whether life-sustaining therapy should be withheld. Thus whilst many doctors would argue that maintaining a persistent vegetative existence does not meet medical goals, if society is to accept that PVS patients should forgo life-sustaining therapy, it must be based on a clear understanding of the facts appertaining to each case and resolution of the moral issues.

A second contestable value-laden use of the term 'futile', argue Crawford and Gostin, is when doctors regard certain forms of treatment as being harmful to the patient. For example, performing CPR on a terminally ill patient who would recover, for a limited period, with gross disabilities. Whilst a decision to withhold CPR may be clear from a medical standpoint, it actually opens up the long standing moral debate on whether a short pain free existence is better than a longer but painful life. This is an issue that cannot be resolved by appeals to medical facts alone; it is a value judgement.

The third application of futility cited by Crawford and Gostin involves a situation where the patient is utilizing scarce medical resources which, some health-care personnel maintain, ought to be available for more needy patients. For example, if providing resuscitative support or intensive care for a patient at the end of her life would deprive other patients of medical intervention. In this case a spurious notion of futility could be employed to mask a covert policy of health-care rationing, when rationing and its pros and cons should be debated on its own terms. Criteria for futility should not, therefore, be driven by cost-containment measures. Even if resources were infinite there would still be a pressing moral need for a judgement that therapy was futile, which should be based on an idea of the patient's best interests as determined by the patient's known values clearly expressed and professional standards.

Futility and Professional Values

The term 'futility' covers many different ethical agendas. Once 'medical futility' is invoked doctors, so it would seem, have authority to override the wishes of patients, families or surrogates; they may take non-treatment decisions without seeking consent or even raising the matter for discussion with a patient. It is often argued that futility judgements by doctors should include the authority to limit a patient or surrogate's choice of treatment, especially with regard to CPR in adults, low birth weight neonates and for fluid resuscitation for severely burned patients. The argument would then be about whether or not relatives should be informed of a futility decision. It might be held that if the alternative to the withholding of therapy is futile therapy then there is no point in either informing the patient or surrogate or even offering a choice. On this view, says Marshall B. Kapp: (1994:172) 'Offering the patient or surrogate an apparent choice when there is no meaningful choice would be as futile as the intervention itself'. Yet unilateral judgements are prone to the criticism that they indicate lack of respect for patient autonomy and dignity, signalling a return to full blown physician paternalism. Thus it may be advisable to discuss the decision with patients but, on the view expressed here, it is of no benefit to the patient to be offered futile therapy. A more modest view, considered by Kapp is that whilst medical futility is determined by the physician, in the interests of honest communication, she should share with the patient or surrogate any information about rejected interventions and her professional reasons for rejecting a particular therapy. This need not limit the doctor's professional right to withhold futile treatment and would conform to the principle of limited paternalism in that doctors acted as moral agents in their view of a patient's best interests whilst acknowledging respect for their autonomy.

Strictly speaking, however, communication about futile therapy is not about respect for patient autonomy and, from a logical point of view a discussion about futile alternatives is pointless. But ethics differs from logic - in the sense that the term 'logic' has been used here - in that a purely logical course of action is sometimes incompatible with our moral expectations of fellow human beings. It is a frequent complaint that health-care professionals are 'too logical' in their approach, and forget that emotional displays are an essential part of human interaction. A display of sorrow when therapy is futile, of course, will bring no physical benefit to the patient but its absence leaves it possible to draw the conclusion that the professional does not care. Without some display of emotion communication of futility judgement may lack sincerity. Words are never enough, for they can always be uttered without sincerity.

A strong view of medical paternalism would, however, maintain that futility judgements are primarily value free and strictly dependent upon medical knowledge. However, the assumption of value neutrality inherent in some appeals to medical futility cannot be sustained. M.Z. Soloman, for example, (1991, 1992) has raised questions regarding the frequent resort to the value-neutrality of medical futility in her research on medical decision-making on life and death issues, and points out that: 'Almost invariably, when futility arguments were involved, they were used to support evaluative judgements based on quality-of-life considerations'. (Soloman, 1992:1239) This, however, introduces a further moral and philosophical question: is futility a workable clinical concept, or is it so permeated with value judgements that doctors should defer to patients and their surrogates? Or, perhaps, there is a third way, whereby it is recognised that futility is a value-laden concept, but is primarily bound up with professional values?

One of the main objections to the appeal to futility decisions is to be found in cases where it is believed that the doctor is responding to a value judgement about the quality of life rather than a clinical fact. But even if we acknowledge that the doctor has made a value judgement this need not be a reason for rejecting the doctor's authority when proposing limitations to therapy, as all limitations to therapy - including non-ventilation of corpses and refusals to perform high risk surgery for minor health problems - involve a value judgement. According to the arguments presented by Tom Tomlinson and Howard Brody (1990) in their assessment of futility decisions in the context of withholding CPR, not even 'physiologic futility' is a value free notion. 'Even the most doomed CPR attempt might have symbolic or psychological significance for the patient or family, who perhaps think it spiritually imperative to "never give up"'. (Tomlinson and Brody, 1990:1278) The question is not whether or not doctors should make value judgements; in fact value judgements are an inescapable aspect of their profession. The real question is twofold: first, how they should communicate value judgements, and second how the process by which they reach value judgements can be understood and broadened into a wider informed societal discussion. The point that must be stressed is that the exercise of professional value judgement is, and must be seen to be, distinct from paternalist abuse of power.

Against the objection that futility judgements indicate a lack of respect for patient autonomy and dignity signalling a return to physician paternalism, Tomlinson and Brody (1990:1276) have argued that 'certain sorts of value judgements must be made unilaterally by physicians as part of medical practice'. They maintain that 'futility judgements can be endorsed on non-paternalistic grounds' and that in making such judgements doctors actually enhance patient autonomy. There is no moral requirement, argue Tomlinson and Brody, to provide any treatment that a patient demands; a doctor has a moral obligation to provide treatment that might do some good and refrain from therapy which she believes to be harmful. If the doctor has no moral power to refuse therapy she has no moral power to refuse harmful therapy. If doctors have a moral duty not to harm they must be recognised as having the ability to identify harmful therapy and the moral authority to withhold it. This restraint is justified with reference to professional integrity and respect for patient autonomy. Thus high risk experimental therapy for minor ailments has no justification in the moral parameters of the medical profession. Now it might be argued that many outlandish proposals have a faint possibility of benefitting a patient and that consequently the doctor should let the patient decide. But this would imply that the doctor has no moral values and is merely a supplier of technical services. Yet no professional can practice with reference to wild possibilities and still retain credibility and respect within the profession. According to the arguments of Tomlinson and Brody decisions to withhold from wild possibilities or high risk therapy are derived from a shared value-laden awareness of the state of the art and what counts as a reasonable course to pursue. Such judgements are made against a background of technical knowledge, professional guidelines, and probabilistic calculations. They do not appeal to absolute certainly, nor should they, for such a quest would paralyse medicine. The doctor has a moral authority to make some decisions about the use to which her skills and products of her experience may be put. The scope of this authority may be bounded on the one hand by the prevailing moral climate (for example, doctors should not withhold therapy on racist or eugenic grounds) and on the other hand by values internal to the profession. Thus a patient should not have surgery when there is a high probability that he will die on the operating table.

Once we depart from misleading models of health-care which see health providers as suppliers of technical resources we can recognise that the issue is not whether the doctor takes moral decisions, but which moral decisions must be taken by the doctor. Here it is important to recognise that value judgements involve a social dimension and are not purely subjective outbursts. This reference to a social dimension involves an understanding of what is commonly understood by references to 'reasonable attempts' to provide therapy and 'unreasonable therapy choices'. So what makes a reasonable choice of what is futile? There must be a socially shared understanding of what is meant by a 'reasonable choice' or a 'worthwhile life'. In this context Tomlinson and Brody speak of an urgent need for an 'effective social dialogue, which can ensure that the value judgements that physicians must necessarily make have an adequate social warrant'. (*ibid*:1280)

According to Tomlinson and Brody, futility decisions, when taken by a doctor acting in accord with the moral standards of the profession and society, actually enhance patient autonomy. A patient is not making an autonomous decision if she opts for therapy of which it can be reasonably said to be futile offering no benefit. A doctor who offers futile therapy is not enhancing the scope for autonomous choice but is simply confusing the issue. It has always been necessary to restrict the range of choices open to a patient - offering a range of options which exclude those recognised as futile.

A Moral Dispute

On the 14 December, 1989, an 86 year old American woman, Helga Wanglie, slipped on a rug and broke her hip. In January, 1990, she developed respiratory failure and was intubated at Hennepin County Medical Center. Over the next five months repeated attempts to wean her from the ventilator proved unsuccessful. In May, 1990, she was transferred to an acute care hospital, and by then it was believed that she had severe irreversible brain damage. The doctors discussed with the family the possibility of limiting further life-sustaining therapy. The family resisted and insisted that she be transferred back to the original hospital, where she was diagnosed as PVS, secondary to severe hypoxic-ischemic encephalopathy. Following readmission vigorous treatment continued, with ventilatory support, antibiotics for continuing pneumonia, artificial feeding, and treatment for electrolyte and fluid imbalance. Because of her age, unsuccessful attempts to wean her from the ventilator, and neurological condition, the medical staff viewed her prognosis as extraordinarily poor and recommended withdrawal of ventilatory support. Although the family agreed to a DNAR order, they resisted extubation and insisted that all other forms of therapy be continued. Her husband understood that, in a PVS, she was unaware of herself and surroundings, and that she would never improve, but he said that he 'hoped for the best', insisting that 'only God can take life'. The family's resistance to discontinuation of therapy was partly personal and partly religious, and they repeated that Helga Wanglie would not want anything done to shorten her life. None of the medical facts were disputed, and the cost of care was covered by a private insurance plan.

Following several family conferences, noting the family's determination that therapy should be maintained, the hospital sought the court's approval for the appointment of a conservator to represent the patient and decide whether continued therapy was appropriate. The hospital's case was that further therapy was *futile* and that the family cannot *demand* that doctors continue therapy which they do not believe to be in the patient's best interests. (Cranford, 1991; Rie,1991; Ackerman, 1991) On 1 July, 1991, Justice Patrick Belois denied the hospital's petition, and appointed her husband as guardian, who had previously indicated his intent to continue treatment. (*Re Helga Wanglie*, 1990) She died, on the ventilator, 5 July, 1991.

This case demonstrates that doctors are moral agents, and that they are prepared to resist therapy which they regard as futile. This matter is particularly acute in decisions about PVS patients, where doctors insist that life-prolonging therapy - including nutrition and hydration - is futile. The appeal to futility places a limit upon patient autonomy: life-sustaining therapy can be refused, but it cannot be demanded. Of crucial importance in these debates is the nature of futility. In *Wanglie* the hospital insisted that continued ventilatory support was 'medically inappropriate', which meant that the patient was unlikely to recover, it would not alleviate her suffering, or enable her to lead a more enjoyable life. The family did not dispute this. The dispute was not about medical facts but an ethical clash between two assessments of the quality of her life; it was not a question of whether or not further ventilation would prolong her life, but an ethical dispute whether her life was worth prolonging, and no appeal to medical expertise alone could resolve it. Further medical facts might have influenced either party to the dispute, but the way forward would have to be based on a resolution of the ethical conflict. In the event of a stalemate a presumption in favour of maintaining life would seem to have been the best likely course in this case, as the distress to the family by her death in such circumstances is likely to outweigh any distress suffered by medical staff who are obliged to provide therapy which they have determined to be of no value. Termination of life-prolonging therapy against family wishes could leave them feeling that her life had been shortened by a conspiracy of professionals and would contribute to a distancing between the medical profession and the public. Appeal to the principle of patient autonomy could also tilt the balance in favour of continued therapy, argues Cantor, (1993:95) who advocates advance directives as a means of settling such disputes: the family's decision, based on known wishes of the patient for continuous life support, he argues, 'should prevail over the physician's judgement about the pointlessness of continuous care.'

These considerations should tilt the balance in favour of continuing therapy in certain cases, despite the genuine unease which doctors face when obliged to maintain therapy which they find morally objectionable. What must be acknowledged, however, is that the doctor's reluctance to provide life-prolonging therapy is very largely a moral one, and this should be recognised and not disguised with references to seemingly value-neutral expressions like 'medically inappropriate'. When appeals to medical futility are made they convey a sense of scientific objectivity, but in reality they may conceal contestable value judgements.

Futility and Autonomy

Over the past ten years or so the medical profession and cost-conscious governments - possibly from different motives - have been very comfortable with the growing momentum in favour of patient autonomy. This is part of the new and wider ethos of citizenship, in which charters expressing dubious commitments to consumer-sovereignty proliferate. But autonomy has been primarily located in the right to say 'no more', and great efforts have been made by the media, as well as the community of bioethicists, to defend the patient's right to refuse life-sustaining therapy. Thus spurious appeals to autonomy have been made in order to give an inkling of sense to the judgement that someone would be 'better off dead' (whatever death is it is not something where one is either better or worse off) and autonomy has been invoked as a means of blurring distinctions between assisted suicide and the right to forego invasive life-prolonging therapy.

In a general atmosphere of concern about over-treatment many authorities have drawn up guidelines for withholding various forms of life-sustaining health-care on the grounds that autonomous patients regard them as futile. But a recent side effect of the autonomy movement, notes Troyen A. Brennan, (1992) is the assertion of physician autonomy; that is, the withholding of therapy because the doctors regard it as futile. This, according to Brennan, (1992:336) is an 'unexpected extension of the right to die'.

Now the notion that patients can forego life-sustaining therapy is justified by appeals to autonomy and privacy and also freedom from unwanted bodily intrusion. As such it is not necessarily related to the right to die. Thus a doctor who withholds life-sustaining therapy on the instructions of a patient, despite her willingness to provide it, is not implicated in the death of that patient. (Lamb, 1987) Quite clearly a doctor's appeal to professional autonomy may give rise to conflict with patients, relatives and surrogates. Doctors may take refuge in medical futility in order to recover the notion of objectivity and scientific rationality, especially in the face of what they see as idiosyncratic or irrational choices by patients and their families. The appeal to medical futility may then enable doctors to believe that their decisions are free from emotional factors. It should be noted in this context that many doctors still confuse the term 'emotional' with 'moral'.

There is a view, no doubt held by many members of the medical profession, that greater patient autonomy actually means less professional authority and consequently the appeal to medical futility is a means of tipping the balance of power back in the direction of the medical profession. But this view is dispelled by Ann Alpers and Bernard Lo (1992:327) who point out that it rests on a mistaken assumption that 'power in the doctor-patient relationship is a zero sum game'. In contrast advocates of informed consent and patient autonomy have pointed out that informed decision-making by patients and their families does not diminish the authority of the doctor and her ability to practice good medicine, but rather facilitates an atmosphere of trust and respect which provides a moral framework within which good medicine can be practised.

As a moral agent the doctor does need some form of appeal to futility as a defence against families who, despite advice and counselling, may insist on medically unjustified therapy which could amount to the torturing of terminally ill patients. This is clearly a problematic area as there are always borderline cases and room for disputes between what the doctors see as futile and what the relatives see as futile. In cases, such as the dispute over Helga Wanglie's continued ventilation, some kind of compromise is required between the competing demands of the relatives for life-prolonging therapy and the moral duties perceived by the doctors to limit medically futile therapy. Such a compromise finds expression in a doctrine of limited paternalism proposed by John Saunders (1994) who argues that the authority which society bestows upon doctors in order to promote health also carries a moral obligation to recognise and withhold futile therapy. Thus:

> In licensing doctors to go about their business, society implicitly entrusts the physician to promote health and relieve suffering. A useless or harmful treatment does not achieve this end. If the aim of medicine is health and health is a form of beneficence, then no individual patient can have a right to a useless or harmful (i.e. maleficent) treatment. (Saunders, 1994:84)

On this view the doctor possesses the moral authority to withhold therapy which is truly believed to result in greater harm than benefit, and that society, which recognises the moral nature of medical practice, empowers doctors to act as moral agents. Thus many doctors would have increasingly serious ethical objections to administering CPR to patients with widely metastatic cancer or septic shock, despite the patient's known preference for survival.

Conclusion

The concept of medical futility, with few exceptions, is value-laden. Yet good medical practice requires that doctors, as moral agents, recognise and resist the employment of futile and maleficent therapy. The fact that futility is a value-laden concept does not negate its value: medicine *is* and ought to be a value-laden profession and its scientific judgements *are* and should be value-laden. Consequently doctors should not refrain from making value judgements. The argument for limited paternalism bridges the alleged incompatibility between the competing claims of patient and physician autonomy; that is, the doctor's expertise gives a degree of moral authority to limit treatment and define futility whilst carrying an obligation to respect the autonomous interests of the patient. The basis for patient autonomy rests on a degree of harmony with physician autonomy for which both parties should strive. This in turn requires the recognition that a doctor is not just a supplier of goods to an indifferent consumer, but that the doctor has a moral authority which is based on the maintenance of a relationship of trust with the patient.

VI Nutrition and Hydration

Introduction

The moral justification for advance directives is the right not to have unwanted therapy inflicted on those who have clearly and autonomously indicated such a preference. In many cases advance directives are an understandable response to the threat of unlimited technical prolongation of life. The question that will be addressed here is to what extent is the provision of nutrition and hydration a form of therapy that a rational agent or surrogate could legitimately forego and to what extent is it a form of therapy that a doctor as moral agent could withhold or withdraw on the grounds of futility?

Is Nutrition and Hydration a Form of Therapy?

A statement adopted by the Executive Board of the American Academy of Neurology in April 1988 maintained that 'The artificial provision of nutrition and hydration is a form of medical treatment and may be discontinued in accordance with the principles and practices governing the withholding and withdrawal of other forms of medical treatment'. The American Medical Association (1986) have defined artificial nutrition and hydration as a 'life-prolonging medical treatment', thus endorsing a general consensus in law and medicine that artificial nutrition and hydration is a form of medical treatment that can be withheld. In 1991 the Institute of Medical Ethics in the UK published a majority view that 'it could be morally justified to withdraw artificial nutrition and hydration from patients in persistent vegetative state.' It is argued that the provision of nutrition and hydration is a medical rather than a nursing procedure because medical judgement, skills in the insertion of a nasogastric tube, and monitoring are bound up with its management.

There are some dissenting voices. In the United Kingdom the

Royal College of Nurses expressed concern to the House of Lords Select Committee on Medical Ethics (1994:18) that they 'see feeding somebody as very fundamental to our whole practice and that the withdrawal of feeding, in whatever form it is being given, can produce very strange conflicts for us.' Case law in the USA, and emerging legal opinion in the UK, however, reveal a strong acceptance of the principle that patients or their surrogates should have the right to refuse therapy, including nutrition and hydration. There is also an emerging consensus that requests for patient transfers from staff who find this morally unacceptable are inappropriate.

A continuum of feeding methods runs from natural breast feeding to mouth feeding and serious invasive procedures which may require surgical intervention. At which stage does feeding become treatment? In the case of Claire Conroy, who was being fed by means of a nasogastric tube, the trial court granted permission for the tube to be removed but the finding was appealed and reversed because the Court of Appeal held that death following the removal of the feeding tube would be due to dehydration and starvation, which implied active killing. However, the Supreme Court of New Jersey reversed the appellate decision, arguing that a nasogastric tube was a form of maintaining life by mechanical means and was akin to a ventilator. Hence, the court argued, the tube was a form of therapy, which the patient/surrogate had a right to refuse.

This argument reveals the emergence of a distinction between natural and artificial modes of feeding of which it is extremely hard to be precise. The best that can be said is that a nasogastric tube requires some form of medical attention, calling for skill and knowledge.

It is obvious that the distinction between ordinary and extraordinary treatment is not relevant to artificially supplied nutrition and hydration, which does not involve the full range of complex medical technology. Whatever the precise meaning of extraordinary therapy the normal idea is of something involving massive technological intervention. Thus in the case of PVS patients, who are considered as candidates for the withdrawal of nutrition and hydration, the distinction appears to have been redrawn in terms of artificial and natural procedures. Thus in *Cruzan*, Justice William Brennan said:

> The artificial delivery of nutrition and hydration is undoubtedly medical treatment. The technique to which

Nancy Cruzan is subject - artificial feeding through a gastronomy tube - involves a tube implanted surgically into her stomach through incisions in her abdominal wall. It may obstruct the intestinal tract, erode and pierce the stomach wall or cause leakage of the stomach's contents into the abdominal cavity... Artificial delivery of food and water is regarded as medical treatment by the medical profession and the Government. [cited by Aldridge, 1994:17-18]

In *Airedale NHS Trust v Bland* a distinction was also drawn by Sir Thomas Bingham, Master of the Rolls, between artificial and natural procedures where evidence was accepted that 'artificial treatment by nasogastric tube is also medical treatment', and that 'mechanical pumping of food through the tube is a highly unnatural process.'

A similar case occurred (*Frenchay Healthcare NHS Trust v S*) where it was claimed that the reinstatement of interrupted artificial feeding was invasive and not in the patient's interests. This case involved a 24 year old man, known only as S, who had survived a massive drug overdose three years earlier, but was diagnosed as PVS with no prospect of recovery. When, in January, 1994, as the result of an accident, his feeding tube was dislodged, Frenchay National Health Service Trust in Bristol, where the man was being treated, sought the court's permission not to reinstate it on the grounds that this invasive procedure was not in the patient's best interests. The High Court approved and, after considering evidence from several expert witnesses, the Law Lords upheld the ruling that it was 'not in S's best interests for feeding to be reinstated'.

There is, however, a moral dimension to the classification of certain treatments as medical. It is generally agreed that futile medical treatment, where burdens vastly exceed benefits, can be withheld, although the question whether or not the withholding of nutrition and hydration extends beyond medical treatment is still controversial. One way around this controversy is to declare certain therapies medical and thus an extension of medical treatment to include nutrition and hydration would diffuse a moral dilemma. This course is still problematic. Oral feeding, for example, is not something that nursing staff would easily refuse to administer. But why, having accepted the withdrawal of mechanical feeding, is there resistance to the withdrawal of oral feeding if it is of no benefit? Robert Veatch (1993:4) has put forward a hypothetical test case concerning 'a terminally ill, imminently dying patient who has refused medically-supported nutrition and is rendered so uncomfortable by oral feeding that it is refused as well.' Veatch asks whether the arguments used to support refusal of therapy, then extended to medically-supported nutrition, could not also be applied to oral feeding.

It has, nevertheless, been argued that nutrition and hydration is not a therapy, even if it is provided on the instructions of a therapist in a therapeutic environment. Among the differences between nutrition and hydration and medical treatment is the fact that only the latter is withdrawn when the patient recovers. Food is not medicine; it is not comparable to antibiotics or blood-transfusions, and it is somewhat absurd to treat it as such. Medicine is administered as a cure, or relief, for diagnosable pathological conditions. Food is provided to meet the body's need for basic resources. Even when food has some medical significance - for example, to alleviate pain or combat certain deficiencies - this function is indirect. A patient may surprise physicians and live or even recover after the withdrawal of medicine, but will certainly die if food is withheld. If it is maintained that withdrawal of nutrition and hydration is not equivalent to the withdrawal of therapy then the withdrawal of food from patients in persistent vegetative states will be seen as a form of euthanasia, not as a policy of 'treating for dying.' According to this argument, if persistent vegetative state patients are not dying and if they are hungry there is a human duty to feed them. Giving food to the hungry also has an important ethical symbolic role such that those who deny food to the hungry represent a paradigm case of a denial of fundamental human relationships. The revulsion against the denial of food to patients in persistent vegetative states is not based on crude emotion but is grounded in a long-standing moral tradition in which food has a basic symbolic role in the expression of human compassion. What is often overlooked in this objection is that the revulsion against the denial of food is also against the context in which food is withheld. Refusal to feed a starving child is morally abhorrent. But in a caring context it may be difficult to establish malicious intent.

When is it a Duty to Withhold Nutrition?

There are cases when it is clearly humane to withhold food; for example, nutrition may cause pain and discomfort and when the distress caused by feeding outweighs any potential benefit. This is not always easy to accept. Julie Fenton (1994:84) points out how 'The provision of food and water is so important that family, friends and staff need to have someone put it to them that many patients in a terminal situation are not aware of hunger or thirst and that trying to satisfy a supposed hunger or thirst may cause or prolong suffering.' But if it is withdrawn for non-therapeutic purposes and its provision has not been established as futile, then those who authorise this course should state clearly that they are engaged in euthanasia. Although there are strong grounds for the discontinuation of nutrition and hydration in a very late stage in the dying process it might be noted that PVS patients in many cases are stable and their condition is not terminal.

Those who oppose the withholding of nutrition and hydration maintain that withdrawal of nutrition and hydration is not strictly akin to the abatement of useless therapy because 1) in many cases food is not therapy and 2) even when it does not assist in a cure it may still bring comfort. Moreover, they might argue that it makes no difference whether the food is served on a tray, spoon-fed, eaten with the aid of artificial dentures or administered through a tube. It should be noted in this context that a significant proportion of patients in nursing homes for the elderly are kept alive by tube-feeding. The intentional denial of food for non-therapeutic reasons is nothing other than euthanasia. The key problem in PVS cases is whether the technical means of supplying food is a futile intervention. But it is hard to say whether the withdrawal of nutrition and hydration or its continuation is in a patient's best interests when the patient is diagnosed as being in a PVS. In a state beyond the capacity for awareness the patient cannot experience or express interests. Arguments in favour of a decision either way inevitably fall in the direction of the interests of others. This, at least, should be openly admitted.

The significance of withdrawing nutrition and hydration from PVS patients in England was highlighted in the case of *Airedale NHS Trust v Bland*, which involved Anthony Bland, a twenty one year-old man who entered a PVS following the Hillsborough football stadium disaster in 1989. Anthony Bland was 17 years old at the time of the disaster and had not given prior indication of his wishes should he find himself in such a condition. Following a two year long legal campaign by the hospital authorities, supported by Bland's parents, the plea for the withdrawal of nutrition and hydration was upheld by Sir Stephen Brown, the President of the Family Division of the High Court, who ruled that doctors would not be acting illegally if they discontinued life-sustaining treatment in order to end Mr. Bland's 'living death'. This ruling was upheld by the Law Lords in February, 1993. Its effect is to protect doctors from the possibility of criminal prosecution for murder if they go ahead and discontinue life-supporting therapy. According to Sir Stephen Brown his doctors 'may lawfully discontinue and need not afterwards furnish medical treatment except for the sole purpose of enabling Mr. Bland to end his life and die peacefully with the greatest of dignity and the least pain, suffering and distress'. In this particular ruling all judges agreed that the case revolved around the patient as subject and that no other considerations were deemed relevant. The medical facts were beyond dispute: Anthony Bland's condition was irreversible. The cost of therapy did not play a determining role; no complaint was made by the caring authorities concerning the allocation of resources to Mr. Bland. Whilst the views of relatives were considered, they were not deemed to be of primary importance. The ruling, however, coincided with the wishes of relatives in this instance but it did not address future potential cases where the relatives disagreed with the doctors. However, a case occurred in November, 1994, which involved a dispute between close family members with regard to the withdrawal of nutrition and hydration. It concerned a 28 year old man who was a victim of a motorcycle accident in 1991 which left him in a PVS. The young man, known as Mr. G., remained in a PVS until the hospital caring for him applied for the withdrawal of artificially supplied nutrition and hydration. Whilst his wife supported the application his mother contested it. Nevertheless the Judge, Sir Stephen Brown, President of the High Court Family Division, ruled that it was in the man's 'best interests' that he be allowed to die. (*Mail on Sunday*, 27 Nov:16-17) This particular ruling, so it would appear, tilts legal opinion in support of the hospital authorities in cases where there is no clear prior choice by the patient and the family is divided.

The Bland ruling was, despite a lack of clarity regarding future cases involving a contest of interests, significant in English law and medical practice. The Law Lords made it clear that the provision of an advance directive should be determinative. The ruling also allows doctors to withdraw life-sustaining therapy from patients who have not given an advance directive and it concedes that nutrition and hydration are forms of therapy and decisions to discontinue them is a 'clinical matter'. It should be stressed that if it is established that nutrition and hydration supplied to PVS patients is a form of therapy which doctors no longer have a duty to provide once it is considered futile, then the subsequent and inevitable death of the patient cannot be regarded as euthanasia or unlawful killing. No doctor has a duty to persist in the employment of futile therapy and cannot be morally responsible for the patient's death if the therapy is withheld. The crucial ethical issue concerning the withdrawal of nutrition and hydration is *not* about acts or omissions (whether omitted actions such as withholding food are the same as actions to bring about death) but whether or not nutrition and hydration constitute a form of futile intervention.

Whilst the Law Lords made it absolutely clear that the ruling in *Bland* was not a step in the direction of euthanasia or doctor assisted suicide, in the media it was not clearly separated from euthanasia proposals, and it gave the pro-death movement a great boost, bringing out all the cliches about 'death with dignity'. An editorial in *The Guardian* (20 Nov., 1992) compared the *Bland* ruling with another case involving a doctor who was convicted of attempted murder after administering potassium chloride to a terminally ill cancer patient, and described the BMA's distinction between withdrawal or withholding therapy and a lethal injection as 'philosophical nonsense'. In general the *Bland* ruling was wrongly reported as a step forward towards the legalisation of voluntary euthanasia and the 'right to die with dignity', despite the fact that the patient was unaware of any such rights and had not issued an advance directive. Anthony Bland died on Thursday, 4 March, 1993. The *Bland* ruling raises several questions. Despite massive media approval of the 'right to die with dignity', this right was not exercised by the patient, but by the doctors supported by the parents. It gives legal protection to medical decisions based on the doctor's beliefs concerning the quality of life, and whilst the actual decision to withdraw nutrition and hydration was based on a belief that it was in the patient's best interests, it is questionable whether this is a step in the direction of further patient autonomy.

The problem in *Bland* was that discussion of futility was overlaid with references to it being in the patient's best interests to die. This was highlighted by the fact that withdrawal of nutrition and hydration would inevitably lead to death. In a written Memorandum to the House of Lords Select Committee on Medical Ethics, Dr. Sophie Botros (1994:23) expressed her misgivings.

> ...one of the main reasons for moral unease in the Bland case is the inevitability of this termination of life (by food withdrawal), when it cannot even be claimed to be in the patient's best interests since he is permanently insensate. The claim that it is at least *not* in the patient's best interests *to continue* with life-sustaining treatment does not seem a sufficient moral justification for what

appears, as a result of the above consideration, to be morally undistinguishable from deliberate killing.

On this argument it would appear that the criteria for withholding futile therapy is indistinguishable from the intention to bring about the patient's death. This is what is unsettling in decisions to withhold nutrition and hydration from PVS patients.

In Scotland there have been no prosecutions of doctors who, with the relatives' permission, withdraw food from patients for whom they decided that further treatment is futile. In most cases this is negotiated skilfully with relatives, but there are still some problematic cases. In one case the doctors were resisted by the mother of a twenty four year-old man, Stuart Paterson, who had been in a PVS for four years following an accident. His mother claimed that he had made 'enormous progress', that he could blink 'yes' and 'no', move his limbs and make body movements on request. She told the *Telegraph* (20 November, 1992) that he 'prefers sport on television and likes people chatting to him all day'. Despite the doctor's advice the family raised £35,000 to pay for his care in the Royal Hospital and Home in Putney, London, a leading unit for attempts to rehabilitate PVS patients, before taking him home in June, 1991. In another Scottish case doctors at the Glasgow Royal Infirmary proposed withdrawal of food to a PVS patient, Bruce McLeod, whose mother initially agreed but asked for a postponement for a further two months. Her minister, the Reverend Alexander Green, who was closely connected throughout McLeod's treatment, said in *The Guardian*, 20 November, 1992: 'Finally she reluctantly agreed that this was the best way forward. Afterwards she was pleased and felt it was the right thing'.

Fears have been expressed that pressure will be put on relatives of PVS patients to agree to the withdrawal of nutrition and hydration. The parents of another Hillsborough victim, who at the time of the court's ruling in *Bland* was also in a PVS, were believed to have gone into hiding to avoid reporters from the gutter press who repeatedly knocked on their door asking if they wanted their son's nasogastric tubes removed. Dr. Keith Andrews, Medical Director of the Royal Hospital and Home, expressed his fears over the *Bland* ruling. 'A lot of people have been worried that I was going to come in after the court and say I'm going to stop feeding the patients. The other thing is will the health authorities cease my funding because withdrawal of feeding is now the done thing with PVS?' (*The Guardian*, 20 November, 1992) One of Dr. Andrews' patients, a victim of brain damage after anaesthetic error, was diagnosed as PVS, but now 'smiles to command, laughs at cartoon, shows appreciation for his wife when she comes and cries when she goes'. (*ibid*)

There are problems which arise when it is argued that further nutrition and hydration is both futile and against the best interests of a PVS patient. In *Bland* Lord Goff argued in favour of discontinuation of nutrition and hydration and implicitly linked the futility of providing nutrition and hydration to 'best interests'. Referring to 'overwhelming evidence that, in the medical profession, artificial feeding is regarded as a form of medical treatment', Lord Goff said:

> But in the end, in a case such as the present, it is the futility of the treatment which justifies it's termination. I do not consider that, in circumstances such as these, a doctor is required to initiate or continue life-prolonging treatment or care in the best interests of his patient.

Their Lordships agreed that in a normal doctor-patient relationship feeding was a necessary duty to sustain life. But in *Bland* they held it was of no benefit to the patient and therefore there was no duty to continue feeding. In this case the criteria for futility was therapy that is 'not in the best interests of the patient' and if this were established there was no duty to feed. But in the case of a PVS it is not easy to determine what the best interests actually are. Normally 'best interests' are calculated with reference to a predicted balance of burdens and benefits, but in the proposal to withdraw nutrition and hydration there is nothing to calculate; the patient will be dead. What is being weighed up is life versus death. So, it would seem, that criteria for futility in such cases cannot be determined with reference to best interests. Moreover, in a PVS the patient is unaware of either the benefits and burdens of continuing therapy and consequently cannot be said to have any interests. What appears to be the case in the Lords' deliberations in *Bland* is that 'having no interests' was implicitly linked to 'having no interest in further therapy' and hence to it being in the patients 'best interests' to have therapy discontinued. But a physical state in which a patient cannot be said to manifest any interests is simply that; it is undetermined. One may infer that 'having no interests' means equally having no interest in either the continuation or discontinuation of therapy.

This position might be remedied, however, with a concept of 'best interests' which was determined by the patient rather than by medical opinion. For example, a person might have an image of bodily integrity which precluded continuous existence in a PVS as an object of pity. A person might also have an altruistic desire not to be the cause of a prolonged ordeal for one's family. These reasons were cited by the Law Lords in *Bland* in favour of the withdrawal of nutrition and hydration but they cannot be derived from objective medical facts as they are part of the patient's subjective beliefs.

VII Therapy Abatement When Treatment is Expensive

Introduction

This chapter seeks to maintain an ethical distinction between autonomous refusal of therapy and cost-containment policies. A further separation is also argued for between cost-containment policies and criteria for the beneficent withholding of futile therapy. Whilst the maintenance of these distinctions is considered ethically important it is not suggested that policies aimed at reducing health-care costs lie beyond the scope of ethical investigation. Some proposals, including health-care rationing are examined. The primary purpose here is simply to insist that the principle of limited paternalism - respect for patient self-determination limited by professional awareness of a patients best interests - is morally separate from a doctor's role as custodian of the public purse.

Autonomous Refusal and the Cost of Therapy

Demands for greater patient autonomy reveal a desire by individuals to achieve greater levels of self-management against professional paternalism and bureaucracy. Yet in much of the literature of recent bioethics support for autonomy has become an ideology which many approve of without reflection on the range of choices that can be freely sought by an individual. Most discussions, for example, focus on the autonomous refusal of therapy, reflecting fears of over-treatment. This is how autonomy has been championed by euthanasia societies. It is easily forgotten that the greatest problem for the majority of the world's population is that of under-treatment. Even in the wealthiest countries health-care resources are too thinly stretched to provide all of the population with adequate care. At present thirty seven million Americans have no health cover; forty five million are under insured. Opinion surveys on the reluctance to donate organs reveal that fears of under-treatment ('the doctors might give up before I'm really dead') is one of the main reasons for not carrying donor cards. As a corrective to the view that large-scale public-opinion support for treatment abatement is an indication of support for euthanasia it might be suggested that such demands are simply part of a wider movement in favour of more control over a whole range of informed therapy options, which are not reducible to slogans concerning the 'right to die'.

It is sometimes argued that a patient should have the right to refuse therapy - and possibly life-prolongation - on the grounds that it is too costly, or burdensome on relatives, to continue. This, however, is not a question of autonomous choice as the conditions under which the choice is expressed may present the agent with a situation over which she has no sense of free choice whatsoever. Some disabled people may exercise their 'right' because of lack of adequate services, support and money. Given a free choice few people would opt for circumstances in which financial restrictions limited their range of free expression. Moreover, the cost of therapy should be recognized as a social or political problem with a collectivist solution. A situation in which a patient dies in a state of anxiety over payment for therapy can be seen as an immoral outcome of a society which has adopted a restricted, distorted and abstract individualist perspective.

Advocates of medical cost-containment have recently identified autonomous refusal of life-sustaining therapy with programmes designed to scale down the alleged escalating cost of health-care. Some US advocates of medical cost-containment see a direct link between the fourteenth amendment right to refuse medical intervention and financial savings. Given the amount of pressure to import US models of health-care provision into the UK the following proposal by K.K. Fung (1993) should be regarded as cautionary. Fung maintains that 'If the patient is offered compensation to give up his *de facto* right to aggressive treatment, insurance premiums can be reduced' (1993:275) Moreover, if physician-assisted suicide were made legal then insurance schemes involving physician-assisted death with benefit conversion could also be introduced. Fung (1993:276) thus proposes a two pronged incentive scheme to 'curtail over treatment and the spiralling health-care costs in major illnesses.' The scheme would involve a synthesis of benefit conversion for early termination of treatment and a 'dignified death.' Thus 'by offering the right to die with dignity, an escape valve to the current fiscal over-commitment and concomitant human suffering is created.' (*ibid*:279) Fung's two pronged approach 'ensures that the system would not be abused when private and public entitlements are converted into death benefits, there is no danger that the terminally ill would spend their converted benefits and then refuse to die. And since the healthy elderly cannot easily disguise themselves as terminally ill, there is also no danger of massive influx of volunteers to overwhelm the conversion system.' (*ibid*:283)

Fung also considers the potential benefit of policies which simply encourage an early death without compensation. Surely this would save even more resources. Fung rejects this and stresses the importance of giving consideration to the wishes of volunteers and their opinions on what should be done with the money saved. One might, for example, save money on some patients only to squander it on 'more futile treatment for those who should have chosen, but refuse to choose, dignified death.' (Fung, 1993:283) Early deaths save funds. If this can be harmonised with programmes for physician-assisted death through compensation then everyone stands to gain, argues Fung, who cites surveys showing that '46% of health-care costs in the last year of life are spend in the last 60 days' (*ibid*:283-4) and that '25-35% of Medicare expenditures go to only 5-6% of those enrolees who will die within the year.' (*ibid*:287) With these kind of financial incentives to encourage patients to opt for death are we not in danger of sliding into a slippery slope where the 'right to die' becomes a 'duty to die?' Fung (*ibid*:286) dismisses the objection that pressure will be put on the terminally ill to die. He points out that people with rights always get pressured to use them. Yet many choose not to. People are put under pressure to vote, but many choose not to. However, the terminally ill belong to a different category than the political abstainers. In one important respect they are weaker and more prone to succumb to pressure. Fung's response to the slippery slope objection is unhelpful; the world, he says, is full of slippery slopes. (*ibid*:287)

Among the problems with Fung's attempt to reduce the ethically based right to refuse therapy to an asset of value are 1) the problem of inegalitarianism; the poor would be the first to choose an early death. 2) Medical problems would also emerge in relation to the patient's prognosis. Compensation schemes for physician-assisted death would, presumably, be operative on terminal patients. Can the patients and their doctors be absolutely sure that they are dying? It might be noted that the longer the delay in reaching certitude the less savings there would be from treatment curtailment. 3) There would also be administrative problems: when should payment begin? If payment is made before death at what point is it to be made effective? If payment is made after death then it would appear to be little different to any other form of insurance. These questions are raised by George Dellaportas (1993) in a reply to Fung. Dellaportas also raises an extremely important question which must apply to many schemes for medical cost-containment: Why should savings be made out of the patients? Why not contain the expenditure of the massive health-care bureaucracies? In this context Dellaportas (1993:290) cites surveys which indicate that 'One in every 4 or 5 dollars spent on health-care now goes to administrative costs, mostly to support a monstrous bureaucracy and highly paid executives.' He notes how: 'A 1991 Harvard study found that between "19.3 and 24.1% total spending on health-care" in the US represents administrative costs.' It would seem prudent to consider cost-containment policies in this area. According to Dellaportas (1993:290) these figures translate to 'between 200 and 250 billion dollars for the 1993 health-care bill of almost one trillion dollars, enough to balance even the annual federal deficit.'

Rather than taking directives from US apostles of cost-containment at the patient's expense and the reduction of ethical rights to disposable assets it is advisable to reinsist on what is valuable in the principles of equal access to health-care found in the National Health Care Systems of Canada and Germany, both of which have a higher proportion of aged citizens yet much less *per capita* health-care costs. (Dellaportas: 1993:290)

Health-Care Rationing and Medical Futility

Arguments about the cost of therapy are frequently introduced in the context of discussions concerning the alleged futility of a proposed form of treatment. But is an appeal to medical futility an appropriate way to solve the problem of allocating scarce medical resources? Doctors play an important role in the allocation of resources and have accepted their role as distributors of society's expenditure on health-care. Scarcity may involve a lack of funds for new equipment, hospital beds or drugs, or even a shortage of organs for transplantation. Whilst the rationing of health-care is widely practised there have been few political initiatives in this area and, as a general rule, decisions regarding under-treatment are left to doctors. This is usually justified with reference to principles which refer to patient's needs and potential benefits which doctors have expertise in recognising. In this context health rationing is frequently overlaid with references to medical futility: hence expensive cardiac surgery may be withheld from a patient on the grounds that such therapy would be futile if offered to a heavy smoker. Underpinning the decision here is an awareness of limited resources. Yet frequently the decision to withhold therapy is defended by an appeal to medical futility. This is both disingenuous of doctors and those in authority over the macro-allocation of resources who expect doctors to ration health-care. Decisions to withhold treatment are not morally justified with reference to problems of resource allocation. As Cantor (1993:95) points out: 'resource allocation issues should be resolved by social judgement - as reflected in considerable regulatory and legislative determinations -and not by individual practitioner's judgements that public funds might be better expended elsewhere...' The answer, in principle, is straightforward: doctors should not use futility as a criterion for rationing; rationing is not a matter of therapeutic privilege, and doctors should not allow their expertise to be employed as a buffer for society's unwillingness to meet the full cost of health provision, and openly admit that there are insufficient resources for those who need them. Society should face the dilemma squarely: either provide more resources or devise schemes for rationing. There are unquestionably very serious dilemmas posed by the escalating costs of some forms of therapy. But it is important to maintain a distinction between arguments concerned with an equitable distribution of social resources with arguments concerned with the potential benefits which may be derived from a proposed set of therapeutic procedures. In a statement to the House of Lords Select Committee on Medical Ethics (1994:23) the Department of Health stressed that 'resource allocation has no part to play in discussions concerning the withdrawal of an individual's life-prolonging treatment. The doctor is obliged to do the best he can for the patient under his care.' The BMA also said that medical judgements 'should be made when clinically appropriate, not when funds run out.' (*ibid*:23)

Nevertheless, references to the cost of medical resources have began to surface in many recent ethical decisions and there is a body of opinion which considers that cost should be an important factor when making decisions to withhold or forego life-sustaining therapy. Giles R. Scofield (1991:28) poses the dilemma as follows:

> Our increasing awareness that the limitations of human knowledge, resources, and ingenuity impose finite horizons on medicine's ability to ward off disease, disability, and death has forced us to acknowledge that we must either limit medical intervention on a societal and individual basis or bankrupt ourselves.

One area where criteria for futility are linked with problems of cost-containment and resource allocation is in the consideration of therapy options for the elderly. In a paper which addressed some of the ambiguities in the expression 'not clinically indicated', Tony Hope, David Springings and Roger Crisp (1993) reported on enhanced survival rates for cardiac surgery among the over seventies. But they noted an implicit selection factor among those deemed eligible for surgery. The expression 'not clinically indicated', they point out, has two distinct meanings: first, it means that the operation will not be of overall benefit to the patient, that the high risk of death during the operation outweighs the likelihood of post-operative benefit. Second, it can mean that the proposed operation is not the right allocation of available resources. These two meanings are concealed within the same expression. But the former refers explicitly to the well-being of the patient whilst the latter may contain implicit value judgements about expenditure on the elderly and the general distribution of society's resources.

Allegations that doctors were running together cost-containment decisions with value judgements regarding the elderly and insane appeared in a *Sunday Times* report (9 October, 1994) which claimed that UK doctors in nursing homes for the elderly were conducting a euthanasia policy. The *Sunday Times* claimed that of the 200,000 people in long-stay nursing care in the UK, up to a quarter of them will not receive influenza vaccination during the coming winter. The dilemma was illustrated with reference to a long-stay mental hospital in Fareham, Hampshire, where during the winter of 1993 vaccination was withhold from 17 long-stay mentally disturbed patients: when the virus struck eight patients died during the first week. None of the families in this case were consulted about the decision not to vaccinate.

The problem of health-allocation and its funding is of major importance but the solutions lie ultimately with Governments and the public, who must decide how much of a nation's wealth should be allocated to health resources. An ethicist who simply responds uncritically to dilemmas caused by an inadequate macro-allocation is out of touch with the ethical issues. For example, one of the first questions the philosopher should raise concerns the scarcity assumption which underpins the so-called crisis in health-care allocation. There are wasteful procedures to be tackled, defensive medical practices which lead to unnecessarily expensive treatment, excessive bureaucracy and, above all, a need to re-assess social priorities. Society has to determine the total allocation of resources for health-care, and ethicists who speak uncritically of a need to ration and exclude certain provisions, introducing quality of life criteria into therapy decisions, seem to forget that other services, such as the fire service and the police, are engaged to combat injury and death. Although restrictions may be placed on the overall funding of these services, ethicists are not asked to consider quality of life decisions regarding the recipients of fire service protection and police protection.

It is often argued that criteria for medical futility has a social dimension and that consequently societal concern with the allocation of resources should be considered when deciding whether therapy is futile. For example, it might be argued that respect for autonomy implies a social framework and consequently since citizens have duties as well as entitlements then limits to therapy should also take community welfare into consideration. On this argument autonomy is closely linked to questions of equity and distributive justice. And if personal choice is limited by notions regarding community welfare, criteria for futile intervention should recognise the costs to the community.

This line of reasoning, although superficially attractive, breaks down once we question the linkage between an individual's actual choice and the distribution of resources. If a UK citizen withdrew from all health-care provision the beneficiary would not be other users of the health service or the community, but the treasury. Few individuals, even when acting collectively, have any real influence over the distribution of resources. Proponents of the above argument would appear to believe that individuals in the democratic countries of the developed world exercise some form of direct influence over the distribution of that nation's resources. But this is nonsense: no democracy has yet achieved that level of integration between individuals and the executive in control of the state who determine the overall distribution of welfare. An ability to contribute to a process of 'voting the bounders out' every few years is not enough on which to build a case for establishing a duty to forego costly therapy. By no stretch of the imagination can autonomy be linked to distribution systems over which an individual has little or no control. This is not, however, to argue against a very pressing need for a fair and equitable system of health-care provision, but simply a statement that under existent politico-economic structures there is no link between autonomy and distribution. The appeal to community interests as a limit to therapy is, in effect, a plea to authorise governments to set even further limits to health-care. The objection is twofold: first, there are insufficient democratic restraints on governments; and second, the level of individual care would be even more determined by whatever economic theory was fashionable and reflective of the prejudices politicians hold about social worth.

Age Care Rationing and the Duty to Die

The argument that the elderly have a duty to die and consequently release much needed health-care resources has been put forward most forcibly by Battin (1994) who cites lists of statistics regarding the escalating costs of providing health-care for the elderly. She argues for a change in attitudes whereby the elderly, in a cost-consciousness society, would recognise a time to die and see it as their duty to elect for a quick termination. Battin favours a direct termination of life, rather than gradual abatement of costly therapy, as the most humane and cost-effective solution to the escalating cost of caring for the elderly.

Yet whilst Battin outlines and applauds the moral desirability of such a programme she astutely recognises problems in its implementation. As a minimum requirement a just system of health rationing depends on the functioning of the scheme such that the distributive gains are actually realised and seen to be realised. A failure to provide such a guarantee is the fundamental weakness of all rationing models. Thus Battin provides a double warning regarding the implementation of her age rationing proposal. First:

> the appropriate response to the apparent cost-containment crisis in health-care is not necessarily to devise just policies for enacting rationing, by age or in any way, but to reconsider the societal priorities assigned various social goods...
>
> Second, a redistribution policy cannot be just without adequate guarantees that resources will, in fact, be redistributed as required... Furthermore, a just rationing system requires a background of just institutions to ensure its operation, and neither the United States, nor Great Britain can boast a full set of these... (Battin, 1994:77)

It is the failure to produce, or even show any signs of producing, a just system of redistributing the alleged benefits of a rationing system which reveals the hollowness behind the rhetoric of health-care rationing. Thrift may be desirable in some areas, but it should not be confused with justice, with which it may often conflict. If our society is to engage in a major debate on health-care rationing the parameters of the discussion should include the entire range of social priorities. A public debate which is limited to health-care and the need to contain its costs will, from the start, be a rigged debate and must be exposed as such.

Escalating costs of providing health-care have wrongly created a knee-jerk reaction that draconian systems of rationing will have to be considered for an aging population. There are more promising solutions. Apart from a reconsideration of social priorities there is a need for more reflection on the structure of health-care provision. Whilst there are strong tendencies within the administration of the UK's health service towards US market models and consequent rationing it should be stressed that there is little to be learned from a ramshackle system where almost 40 million have inadequate access to health-care and even the most modest reforms in favour of distributive justice have been blocked by powerful commercial interests. The introduction of an internal market within the UK health service, initially justified as a means of cost-containment with benefits to the sick, has led to demoralisation of health-care staff as well as patients, and a massive consumption of administrative costs by the army of managers which is growing faster than available resources. In a recent criticism of waste accompanying the introduction of financial competition between units of the NHS, Angus Clarke (1995) points out that the cost of information technology required for an internal market in health-care is a political imposition which reduces resources for patients, not to mention time spent by consultants in drawing up business plans when they could be treating patients. 'The focus on money and costs', says Clarke, (1995:117) 'is itself costly, and the atmosphere it creates will damage clinical decision-making'.

There is no dispute that health-care provision is costly and costs will continue to increase. But the images which accompany arguments for cost-containment have played a distortive role. Images of expensive high technological equipment employed on every dying patient, further images of hospitals crammed for years with PVS patients with no hope of recovery frequently cloud ethical discussion concerning therapy for the long-term ill. Can society afford these increasing costs, is the question to which these frightening images direct the appropriate answer. To take one issue and put it in perspective: consider the fears of massive costs for PVS patients when balanced against other social priorities. In written evidence to the House of Lords Select Committee on Medical Ethics, Dr. Keith Andrews (1994:223) pointed out:

On the only day the pound collapsed this country lost enough money to keep all of the PVS patients in the United Kingdom cared for in private care for 2,000 years. This is not to suggest that PVS patients should be the priority if such money was put to NHS use but puts into perspective the size of the financial burden.

Conclusion

Fears of massive over-expenditure on health-care are prone to exaggeration and also rest on a mistaken belief that health-care is akin to a bottomless pit which swallows up resources without any return to society. This is patently nonsensical and betrays ignorance of the way that health-care investment can stimulate new technologies. To give but one example; it is said, from an economic standpoint, great expenditure on an aged population can have little benefit on the economy as a whole. Yet the technology which currently serves to make the working lives of young professionals wretched, throw millions out of work, and produce weapons of mass destruction, could be employed to enhance the lives of the chronically sick, the irremediable, and frail elderly. Gorowitz (1993:92-4) has described the beneficial effects - in morale - which computer games had on residents in a Washington residential home for the elderly, and rightly criticised the computer industry for not recognising the potential market among the elderly sections of society. The elderly and frail, he points out, could have their lives transformed with video-text systems, communications networks, where community centres could be linked to each other. Education programs could be made available on many levels according to level of sophistication and mobility. All of this might require modifications to hardware; not necessarily designed for the speed required in a modern office, but for users with limited dexterity and patience, and software modifications may be required to compensate for sensory deficits. One of the great possibilities of cyberspace technology could lie in this direction. The very old and infirm could benefit, and in turn bring benefit to society, from information technology. So far little has been done to explore the kinds of information technology that would not only improve the quality of life of the disabled and elderly but also reap rich rewards for society. This, however, is not a proposal to put the elderly to work in order to offset the cost of their therapy or to propel them in search of economic independence. In a civilized society the elderly and infirm must be regarded as a dependent in a sense in which dependency is wholly compatible with autonomy and dignity. Appropriately designed information technology could provide a step in this direction, giving freedom and access to a vast range of social activities which have traditionally been denied to older members of society. This is certainly a challenge to the computer industry and to educationalists who have it in their power to enhance the lives of the elderly and frail. Maybe one day some of the bioethicists who have devoted so much effort in showing how lives lacking in certain sensory and cognitive faculties are not worth living might accept this challenge which information technology has posed.

VIII Autonomous Refusal

Introduction

During the past twenty years the principle of autonomy has grown to considerable stature in bioethics and medical law. It has been promoted as a counter to both physician and state paternalism; it is enshrined in the doctrine of informed consent, which extends to minors and the mentally disabled, and is invoked in the refusal of life-prolonging therapy. Requests for the autonomous refusal of life-prolonging therapy have, however, been championed by euthanasia societies, cost-containment advocates, and liberal bioethicists. Mechanisms to facilitate the autonomous refusal of therapy, such as living wills and advance directives, together with health-care powers of attorney, proxies and surrogates, have all been attached to the principle of respect for autonomy. These mechanisms are well-established in US law and have found a foothold in medico-legal practice in the UK. Whilst demands for greater autonomy are to be applauded as part of a broader political insistence upon greater control over one's life, it is important nevertheless to draw attention to some of the pitfalls as well as moral and philosophical problems which can be detected in the formal mechanisms devised to advance autonomous refusal of therapy. The first section will examine the principle of respect for autonomy and consider its limitations. Then the tendency to reduce autonomous choice to therapy refusal will be questioned. In the following section mechanisms, such as advance directives, will be shown to have limitations in their ability to express autonomous refusal. However, this criticism of a formalistic approach to autonomous decision-making in health-care is not designed to undermine the principle of autonomy or to protect physician paternalism but to locate autonomous medical decision-making in a trusting relationship between carer and patient based on mutual respect for the best interests of the patient and the ethical standards of professional health-care.

The Principle of Respect For Autonomy and Its Limitations

For members of a moral community the connection between autonomy and morality is beyond question. This also applies to the principle which requires that one respects another person's autonomy, another person's freedom. This principle is often described as the very bedrock of morality. John Rawls has argued, by means of his appeal to the 'veil of ignorance', that the principle of liberty is the first principle to be accepted by a moral community. Thus: 'each person is to have an equal right to the most extensive basic liberty compatible with a similar liberty for others'. (Rawls, 1971:60)

Although it is firmly established in Western legal traditions the principle of autonomy is a relative latecomer to medical ethics and in many respects it is alien to much of medical practice. Doctors are used to acting in accord with their knowledge of a patient's best interests, and patient autonomy has not been easily accepted. As Robert Zussman (1992:10) argues: ' Not only is it a value alien to medical traditions but it is a value that, when converted to rules and regulations, threatens physician's authority.'

The problem with recent application of the principle of autonomy, however, is not so much the restrictions it places on the arbitrary power of physicians - this aspect is to be welcomed - it is rather the problem of reducing morality to the arbitrary decisions of patients. In fact the tendency to reduce moral decision-making to the maximisation of autonomy has left bioethics on the margins of moral inquiry. Autonomy is not the last word; it is a valuable counter to oppression and professional paternalism, but a free decision is neither necessarily wise nor moral. Making the right decision is not merely a matter of letting the patient/consumer/client decide, for a moral respect for autonomy is concerned with the content as well as the form of the decision.

Respect for autonomy places obligations on the professional and provider of services; at a minimal level it requires the provision of information necessary for an open autonomous choice. This in turn requires decisions on how much information is given, how it is to be presented, how understandable and relevant it is. It requires not only comprehension but understanding in the broader context of its meaning, significance and moral status, as well as the consequences of a particular therapy. To understand a proposal patients and relatives must know how it relates to themselves in a meaningful way. Thus respect should be shown towards a patient's known wishes, values, and religious beliefs. However, the principle of autonomy is not unlimited. Other moral considerations may come into conflict with an autonomous choice. One of the most familiar conflicts is when appeals to autonomy clash with appeals to the principles of non-maleficence and beneficence. For example, the principle of non-maleficence, which stresses the imperative not to cause harm, may limit an autonomous request for a course of therapy with harmful side-effects, and the principle of beneficence, which stresses an imperative to benefit without causing harm, might be cited by a medical team who propose to provide a form of therapy which is contrary to the known wishes of the patient. When the principles of non-maleficence and beneficence come into conflict with an autonomous wish to forego therapy accusations of medical paternalism are frequently made. It is, however, important to recognize that many of these disagreements arise out of conflicts between principles, not as is frequently assumed, out of conflicts with paternalistic authority.

The potential for a clash between autonomy and beneficence can be exaggerated; one can act beneficially towards people by respecting their autonomy, by providing them with more information and so on, and one can maintain a person's autonomy whilst overriding certain wishes in the interests of beneficence, as long as such actions do not undermine the capacity to act freely. For example, treating starvation in a bulimic patient does not impair the capacity to act freely.

Limits to Patient Autonomy

On the liberal market model of self-determination there are no limits to patient autonomy, which can involve a rational assessment of the burdens of benefits of life followed by a decision whether or not one's life is worth prolonging. It is then argued that having made an autonomous decision patients then have the right to receive help in ending their lives by means of either doctor-assisted suicide or passive euthanasia. But this view does not take into consideration the moral views of health-care professionals, and it frequently distorts the nature of decisions taken against a background of challengeable social prejudices. Many of the limits which doctors place upon the self-determination of their patients are related to matters of moral concern which weigh heavily within the professional community. There are, for example, strongly held beliefs in opposition to euthanasia on patient request.

In a recent opinion survey of the variables which compete with physician respect for patient autonomy Terri Fried *et al* (1993:723) found 'concerns about the societal and legal implications of clinical decisions, views of the role of the physician, personal moral beliefs, and concerns about killing patients vs allowing them to die'. Fried *et al* conducted a survey of 392 physicians in the US in order to determine whether they would comply with a hypothetical case of a request for euthanasia from an eighty-year-old patient with terminal metastatic lung cancer. The survey was conducted among a population of one third Catholic, 23% Jewish and 20% Protestant doctors. Of the 256 respondents 98% agreed not to intubate in the face of worsening respiratory failure, 85% agreed to give the patient sufficient narcotics to treat the pain but not to cause respiratory compromise and death; 59% agreed to withdraw ventilatory support if the patient was intubated with no hope of coming off; 9% agreed to prescribe enough sleeping pills that would be lethal if taken at once, but only 1% agreed to give a lethal injection. Those who would comply with the patient's requests cited autonomy as a reason, but those who did not cited ethical and legal concerns, although 28% indicated that they would comply with requests for a lethal injection were it legal. This survey revealed a wide range of physician imposed limitations on patient autonomy, with some prepared to honour requests and others unwilling to honour them. These decisions ranged from the decision to initiate life-sustaining therapy to willingness to administer a lethal overdose. Fried *et al* concluded that the physicians in this representative survey attached significance to a distinction between decisions to withhold or withdraw therapy on the one hand and active euthanasia on the other hand, and that respect for autonomy, is not the sole principle underlying physicians' decisions. They concluded that the goal of the medical profession - 'the naturally given end of health' - is incompatible with euthanasia.

The Reduction of Autonomous Choice To Refusal of Therapy

Appeals to autonomy have dominated recent discussions on health-care ethics yet arguments about choosing therapy have been conducted solely in terms of an individual's ability to express a conscious refusal, or at least indicate in advance a surrogate capable of exercising that choice. In 1992, the Appleton International Conference recommended that in the case of a patient who has lost the capacity to make decisions but has given a valid advance directive to refuse treatment and/or has appointed a representative to make decisions about refusal of treatment, such directives and decisions should be respected by doctors and other health-care workers (Appleton, 1992:6). The Appleton Conference -with some dissenting opinion - also advanced a moral justification of active euthanasia on the appeal to autonomy for severely disabled patients who were not terminally ill. Thus patients who retain a 'decision-making capacity who are severely and irremediably suffering from incurable diseases' ought to receive an 'active termination of life by a medical act which directly and intentionally causes death'. (Appleton, 1992:6)

The concept of autonomy is not always adequately represented in decisions concerning treatment abatement. There is more to the exercise of autonomy than mere refusal. In April, 1986, a 28- year-old American woman, Elizabeth Bouvia, successfully established her right to refuse therapy despite the fact that such a course was life-threatening. She was described as quadriplegic. Except for a few fingers of one hand and some slight head and facial movements she was immobile. In the majority of reports concerning her condition she was said to suffer from degenerative and severely crippling arthritis. She was in continual pain. A tube permanently attached to her chest automatically dosed her with morphine which relieved some, but not all, of the pain and physical discomfort. She had previously sought the right to assisted suicide, requesting care in a public hospital whilst she intentionally starved herself to death, but the courts refused her request. However, when the state of her health declined to the point where she could not be spoon-fed without vomiting and nausea, a drastic decision was taken. Noting the court's ruling against her suicidal intentions, the hospital authorities decided that when her weight loss reached a life-threatening level a nasogastric tube should be inserted, even though it was against her will and contrary to her express instructions. Acting on legal advice Elizabeth Bouvia took her case to the California Court of Appeal where she sought 'the removal from her body of a nasogastric tube inserted and maintained against her will and without her consent by physicians who so placed it for the purpose of keeping her alive through involuntary forced feeding'. (Report of the California Courts of Appeal, 24, April, 1986:1317)

The Court ruled in her favour. In his twenty five page ruling, Associate Justice, Edwin Beach, said: 'She has the right to refuse the increased dehumanising aspects of her condition created by the insertion of a permanent tube through her nose and into her stomach'. (Beach, 1991:49) The question of passive euthanasia or assisted suicide was clearly ruled out when the Court stated that it was immaterial whether or not the removal of the tube caused her death. 'Being competent, she has the right to live out the remainder of her natural life in dignity and peace'. (Report, 1986:1317) Having established her right to forego her life-sustaining therapy, a victory secured after a two year long legal battle, Elizabeth Bouvia decided not to have the tube removed. The real issue was not whether she should live or die but how she could control her destiny.

The court ruling and the media attention which focused on Elizabeth Bouvia's campaign for accelerated death reveal only a fragment of the tragic events leading to her request for the removal of life-prolonging therapy. The question has to be raised: to what extent was Elizabeth Bouvia motivated by a response to her physical condition or by her response to long standing societal prejudice against her physical condition? Paul K. Longmore (1987), a prominent disability rights campaigner, points out that she had faced a life-time of social prejudice and discrimination against the disabled. From childhood she suffered from cerebral palsy, was rejected by her parents, penalised in education and employment when she had struggled to develop a productive life. Her training for a career was further penalised by discriminating Social Security regulations. When she requested physician-assisted suicide in a petition that was rejected in 1986 her disability was not the only reason: there were very severe personal stresses; she had become pregnant and miscarried, experienced separation and divorce proceedings. Yet the three psychiatric professionals brought in by her attorneys simply concluded that it was her physical condition, her disability, which motivated her request for death, and consequently ignored the series of emotional blows. (Longmore, 1987) Having listened to the evidence the judge expressed the hope that Bouvia's case would 'cause our society to deal realistically with the plight of those unfortunate individuals to whom death beckons as a welcome respite from suffering.' (cited by Longmore, 1987:195)

It is important to recognise a distinction between the social background to Elizabeth Bouvia's petition and the issue presented to the courts. The courts were interested in whether a rational decision had been taken (as opposed to an impulsive and emotional reaction) based on a realistic appraisal of her situation. That was how her case was presented. But those who assessed her, argues Longmore, had no experience of disability, and had prejudices that no one who is almost totally paralysed and in need of a respirator can experience a life that is worth living. This prejudice, argues Longmore, (1987:166) is what distinguishes many suicide-rights activists from the interests of the disabled:

...some suicide rights advocates proclaim themselves as pioneers of civil rights of people with disabilities. But these *soi disant* champions of disability rights have been even more noticeably absent while disabled people, including Elizabeth Bouvia, have been struggling to establish their right to live meaningfully and work productively in this society.

In some recent discussions on autonomous refusal of therapy idealised models of autonomy have been borrowed from political discourse and applied to health-care with devastating results. The policy of restoring autonomy to mental patients in the United Kingdom over the past decade is one unfortunate example. Releasing patients from institutional confinement without adequate community support has not enhanced their capacity for autonomy. It could be argued that the eminence of autonomy in recent years has less to do with genuine concern with the liberty of the patient than with the need to restrain costs associated with what some perceive as 'over-treatment' or burdens upon the taxpayer. In the political context liberal individualist values have stressed the freedom of persons from state authority and the restraint of tyrants. But these models of autonomy have entered into medical decision-making without allowing for the fact that they have a very different meaning in the area of health-care. In the political sphere restraint of government has been the hallmark of liberal values. With government withdrawal from public welfare commitments the right to opt out of state-run health provisions has been presented as an extension of personal liberty against paternalistic intervention. But freedom from care and medical intervention is not, in itself, a characteristic of autonomy like freedom from political tyranny. The concept of autonomy means more in the moral sphere. As George J. Agich argues:

> The abstract liberal concept of autonomy has its proper place in the legal political sphere, where protection of individuals from tyranny and oppression by powerful others is rightly defended, but not in the moral life, where a fuller conception is required, one that acknowledges the essential social nature of human development and recognises dependence as a nonaccidental feature of the human condition. (Agich,1990:12)

The goal of autonomy in the provision of health-care, especially in Agich's (1990) account of the needs of patients requiring long-term care, is not reducible to the removal of obstacles and state interference. It may also require a maximisation of options and community support. Dependence is not antithetical to autonomy in the moral sphere, where autonomy might well be compatible with dependence upon a nurse or helper. There has been too much emphasis on resistance to unwanted care and paternalistic abuse with little recognition that, for many patients, including the very young and the old, some form of dependence is the condition upon which autonomous decision-making rests. Agich's analysis of autonomy is important in this respect: although relevant to the political and legal sphere the abstract liberal concept of autonomy should not be uncritically extended into the moral sphere and limits on the ideal should include recognition of 'the essential historical and social nature of persons', especially in 'the development aspects of becoming and being a person'. (Agich,1990:12-13)

Abstract individualism has, however, been frequently imported into health-care from political discourse with the result that appeals to an individual's capacity for autonomous decision-making are frequently made against a background assumption that the individual can be detached from wider social implications. This assumption is also bound up with a form of moral subjectivism in which morality is assumed to be purely determined by an individual's subjective desires. But decisions in favour of therapy abatement are not strictly subjective; they require the complicity of the medical staff which is not a private matter. The decision to abate therapy requires at least two people and a complicit society to make it acceptable.

There are many limits on the right to refuse therapy which are compatible with respect for autonomy. A paradigmatic case here would be a fifteen-year-old anorexic suffering from depression. Should she be allowed to starve herself to death? The answer for some is a resounding no: her condition may be said to prevent an autonomous rational choice. The case of the anorexic patient may, nevertheless, provide an instance of a fateful clash between respect for autonomy and a duty to act in the best interests of a patient. A case was reported in *The Guardian* (10 May, 1994) by Sarah Bosely concerning a 26-year-old anorexic who died within several weeks of her release from a London psychiatric hospital after winning her appeal to the Mental Health Commission Tribunal. Initially the patient, Michaela Kendall, was admitted for therapy under the Mental Health Act, but despite some initial success, she had resisted therapy and sought release from the hospital. Experts in treating anorexia protested that she should not have been released as she was so malnourished that her brain was not functioning properly, and consequently was incapable of formulating an autonomous refusal. Nevertheless, whilst the effects of the illness may impair the ability to make a competent decision consent to treatment, even in the case of minors, may be required in law. In a case involving a refusal of blood transfusion Lord Donaldson MR pointed out that 'Treating [a patient] without his consent or despite a refusal will constitute a crime.' (*Re T*,[1992]) However, he went on to say that in the case of doubt, especially when the situation was life-threatening, the public interest in protecting life would be uppermost and if the individual is to override the public interest he must do so in clear terms. In a similar vein, but emphasising professional duties over abstract individualism, Celia Wells (1994:75) sees an obvious limit to autonomous refusal: 'in the particular case where an emergency urgent intervention is required *in order to save a person's life*, it is unrealistic and probably unreasonable to ask other people, otherwise under a legal and/or moral duty to assist, to stand by.'

The fact that there is more to autonomy than the right to refuse has not been fully appreciated by many philosophers and lawyers who have expended large amounts of energy in arguments for the withdrawal of therapy and accelerated death. That there is more to autonomy than the right to an early death was recognized in a decision reached by the Nevada Supreme Court, following the death of Kenneth Bergstedt in 1991.

Kenneth Bergstedt was a 31-year-old ventilator dependent quadriplegic who was cared for by his father. When facing the imminent death of his father Kenneth petitioned the court for the withdrawal of life-sustaining therapy. But whilst the legal proceeding dragged on Kenneth died in circumstances which suggested that his death had been planned. The toxicology report revealed a high level of barbiturates in his system and the respirator clamp had been unfastened so that he could remove the tube from his mouth. Nevertheless, the Court went on to issue a 'decision' in order to 'provide guidance to others who may find themselves in similar predicaments'. The Court expressed a 'state interest' in preserving life, but recognized that an individual's 'right to decide' will 'generally outweigh the state's interest in preserving life', even if the condition is not terminal. But, most important, the Court required that all competent patients be informed of available health-care alternatives before ending life-sustaining therapy. This is interesting because it maintains the crucial link between therapy abatement and autonomy whilst isolating arguments exclusively based on appeals for the right to an early death. Too frequently autonomy is paraded in slogans bound up with the right to die. The Nevada Supreme Court, in this decision, placed autonomy back in the centre of public interest.

A precedent which might have influenced the Nevada Supreme Court was a ruling by the Georgia Supreme Court on a quadriplegic, Larry James McAfee, who pleaded for the discontinuation of ventilatory support. After winning his case, and repeatedly insisting that he would exercise his right- to-die he was offered residence in various institutions with the intention of making his life more productively tolerable. He consequently chose to remain alive. This case would appear to justify the Nevada decision, as it illustrates that patients who opt for discontinuation may do so without knowing all the options available to them.

The background to the court ruling, however, indicates that social factors, rather than disability, played a role in McAfee's request for an early death. At the age of 34 McAfee was rendered ventilator-dependent after a motor-cycle accident. When his insurance benefit of $1 million ran out and he could no longer employ home attendants he was obliged to enter a nursing home. He then decided that his life was not worth living. He tried to turn his ventilator off but could not stand the feeling of suffocation. He petitioned the courts unsuccessfully for permission to be sedated whilst someone switched off his ventilator. However, he acquired a delay mechanism which would enable him to turn off the ventilator and then allow time for sedation to take effect. The court ruled that this was acceptable and the judgement was based on his rationality and state of disability. The case aroused publicity and McAfee obtained support from disability rights activists. When McAfee reversed his decision it was revealed that what he really wanted was social and economic independence - autonomy - not death. A disability organisation arranged for him to be trained for employment in voice-activated computers. But his Medicare benefits ran out, and Medicaid were unwilling to pay for the nursing costs to meet his needs.

Autonomous Refusal and Advance Directives

The potential for dramatic decision-reversals has not been fully appreciated by the architects of living wills and advance directives. For despite their popularity with the media and the bioethicists it has not been demonstrated that living wills have been enthusiastically accepted by the purported beneficiaries of them. Opinion poll surveys have indicated that few people actually complete them. (Emanuel and Emanuel, 1989) Even when they are made out many physicians are reluctant to follow them.

John F. Robertson, (1991) in a critical commentary on the living will juggernaut, speaks of a distrust and ambivalence among ordinary people and policy-makers. He sees the roots of this distrust in 'conceptual confusions and contradictions that inhere in the use of an advance directive to control a future situation'.(Robertson,1991:7) This might be described as 'the new persons argument'. For example, a healthy person signs an advance directive and some time later succumbs to Alzheimer's disease, with little memory or continuity with her former self. She has no recognition of her friends or family and no awareness or recollection of previous decisions. Should the advance directive signed by her former self be put into effect? It might be said that in such cases involving a radical break in psychological continuity we should recognise that we are confronted with a new person. If so, the former person should not be allowed to harm or cause the death of the new person. Self-determination would no longer prevail as the old self has gone. The former person has gone and will never even know if her wishes were carried out or violated. It might even be said that the best interests of the new person lies in a continuation of life-prolonging therapy. Close friends and relatives may experience the loss of the old person as a catastrophe, but this is not experienced by the new person whose apparent needs are for comfort and nourishment. Such examples indicate a level of conflict between honouring an advance directive issued by an autonomous person and serving the best interests of the incompetent new person. It is not clear, argues Robertson, that a prior directive made by a competent person is the most accurate indicator of a person's interest when she becomes incompetent. There is a different framework in the latter case; the rational standpoint on which the prior decision was made is missing. The values and interests of the competent have no meaning to the incompetent. These interests can be distinct. It is the competent person who does not want to be maintained in an incompetent state; we cannot speak authoritatively of the wishes of the incompetent, which do not necessarily rest on any rational basis. Although it is still the same physical identity the patient's interests may have radically changed. 'Yet the premise of the prior directive', says Robertson, 'is that the patient's interests and values remain significantly the same'. (*ibid*:7) But we cannot know this. What we do have, however, is an increasing number of cases, like Bouvia and McAfee, where a strongly held preference is freely reversed. The difference is that in these cases the authors were competent at the time of the reversal. Merely because incompetent patients cannot express a reversal does not guarantee that their interests remain identical to the competent.

A rebuttal of the new person argument has been put forward by Cantor (1993) who argues that the original terms of an autonomous advance directive should have priority over later considerations. Says Cantor: (1993:27) 'the *potential* changeability of people's feelings should not be a basis to bar future-orientated directives.' Cantor draws a parallel between the living will and other legal dispositions, pointing out that the 'law does not withhold enforcement of future-orientated dispositions of property by will, irrevocable trust, or contract, even though the disposer's inclinations might change over time' (*ibid*:27) The original terms of the advance directive, argues Cantor, should not be overturned without additional evidence indicating a need to revoke them: 'In the context of advance medical directives, it should at least be assumed that a directive maker's wishes persist over time unless there is some showing to the contrary.' (*ibid*:27) Cantor dismisses the objection that one might not be capable of imagining the reality of a future state of incompetency, although he does recognise that it ought to 'impel some serious deliberations (by the declarant) about the content of an advance directive.' (*ibid*:27) These assurances presuppose that an advance directive is properly thought out and drawn up in the context of close cooperation between the doctor and the health-care agent with the possible assistance of experienced counsellors. This procedure will be expensive and time-consuming for medical staff. The advance directive is certainly no substitute for a close doctor-patient relationship.

Yet no amount of counselling and preparation would seem to remove the potential for conflict between personal choice and immediate well-being. Cantor considers two examples which test the limits of advance directives: first, an advance directive specifying no treatment if mentally impaired, but the patient succumbs to mental impairment and, apart from occasional periods of alertness, remains incompetent but enjoying relative comfort in a nursing home. Should this patient be treated for pneumonia? A second example is that of a vitalist who ends up mentally incompetent with extreme pain and suffering with terminal cancer. Should every effort to sustain life be employed?

Or to consider a slightly different example: a person signs an advance directive indicating no therapy in the event of a degenerative condition such as Alzheimer's disease. But in the early stages of the disease the patient requests treatment. Should the directive be disregarded? Suppose it is, and the patient continues to deteriorate: should it always be the most recent decision that is regarded as valid? In these cases should advance directives be revoked or merely suspended?

These problems suggest a need for constant attention to the status of the document in the patient's mind.

One objection to the new person argument may lie in an appeal to the wholeness of the self, where it is insisted that the self has a unity that exists over one's entire life, and that if previously competent persons have a history of preferences and values they should be treated - when incompetent - as still having those values. It might be argued that being competent and being incompetent are stages in the same person's life, and that it is only a metaphorical way of speaking when we say 'she isn't the same person anymore.' If this is the case then it could be said that if we are confronted with a single existence we should place greater weight on decisions taken when competent. This, however, is a weak argument which overlooks the fact that people can change their interests and values throughout their lives. At the very least any course of action based on an appeal to the autonomy of persons must respect their capacity to revise their interests.

It must be acknowledged that society does honour wishes and respects the prior dispositions of those who have lost competence. Losing competence is not a basis for allowing others to do to one as they think fit. It is recognised that a being can be harmed even if the harm cannot be experienced or reflected upon. We do not permit experiments upon incompetent patients. To a certain extent these values towards incompetent patients are similar to the way in which society honours the recently deceased. These values are, as Cantor argues, bound up with notions of post-competent dignity and respect where a prospective personal image is of considerable importance. Sympathy for the person who makes a prior declaration that he or she would not wish to be maintained alive in a post-competent state is a reflection of our respect for the notion of having a life-time mastery of one's body. Yet it is hard to reconcile our respect for self-mastery and the protection of one's image of life with proposals to withhold therapy from a life that is pleasantly senile.

It is this potential for conflict between personal choice and the best interests of the incompetent person which weakens the appeal to autonomy in advance directives which specify abatement of life-sustaining therapy. Admittedly it is difficult to verify or assess the extent of this conflict, as in most of these cases the patient remains incompetent until death. But there is plenty of anecdotal evidence of patients being treated, despite a contrary directive, and then recovering with gratitude.

Perhaps the most informative thing that can be said about advance directives is that they are a device for measuring a person's interests, not an expression of certainty which is a characteristic of the will of a deceased person.

A Presumption in Favour of Life

In cases where doubt emerges concerning autonomous refusal of therapy it is often argued that autonomy is not always the highest virtue, and that autonomous refusal may have to be weighed against a presumption in favour of life, especially in cases involving an alleged change of mind, as indicated by the following borderline example by James F. Childress. (1990:14)

> A twenty-eight-year-old man (who) decided to terminate chronic renal dialysis because of his restricted life-style and the burdens on his family - he had chronic diabetes, was legally blind, and could not walk because of progressive neuropathy. His wife and physician agreed to provide him with medication to relieve his pain while he died and agreed not to put him on dialysis even if he requested under the influence of uraemia, morphine sulphate, and Ketoacidosis (the last resulting from cessation of insulin). While dying in hospital, the patient awoke complaining of pain and asked to be put back on dialysis. The patient's wife and physician decided to act on the patient's earlier request that he be allowed to die, and he died a few hours later.

Childress, who is a proponent of the right to autonomous refusal of life-prolonging therapy, nevertheless argues that he should have been put back on dialysis where it could then have been determined whether he had autonomously revoked his earlier decision. If it was then deemed that his earlier decision was uppermost they could have proceeded with more confidence. 'Present revocation', argues Childress, (*ibid*:14) 'takes priority if it is autonomous.'

Of course if a patient becomes incompetent through dementia and is so demented that he cannot understand the choices offered and the potential consequences of any choice then it is not an autonomous revocation. In such cases, argues Cantor, (1993:85) the prior directive should apply: 'The ravings of a deeply demented patient ought not be permitted to override an advance directive.' Quite obviously Cantor recognises that revocation on these terms would make a mockery of the earlier decision. But a more modest course, involving a temporary suspension of the advance directive, is preferable. Ravings can be interspersed with periods of lucidity which are not always identified by busy health-care staff. A temporary suspension would allow time to consider whether an autonomous revocation was being made, and it would also alleviate the anxieties of health-care staff who are reluctant to withhold treatment from those who require it.

Why is it that there is concern, in cases of this kind, over which decision counts? Surely, both were taken by the agent concerned. One obvious answer is that it is the truly autonomous decision that is being sought. But there is another answer which reveals the importance of a presumption in favour of life in doubtful circumstances: a decision in favour of life-prolongation can always be annulled if it turns out that this was not autonomously desired by the patient, but steps taken to end a life cannot be revoked if it is later believed that this was not autonomously desired.

Conclusion

The movement in favour of greater patient autonomy, expressed in living wills and advance directives, has coincided with dramatic changes in the provision and delivery of health-care whereby the doctor is subject to many other responsibilities than patient care. For example, doctors are governed by economic restraints, a limited choice of speciality consultants, and regulations concerning the prescription of drugs. As medicine becomes more of a marketable commodity it can no longer be assumed that the doctor acts unequivocally as the patient's advocate, and the response of patients and the public is an increasing distrust of experts and health-care professionals. Demands for greater autonomy reflect this distrust and provide evidence that the traditional doctor-patient relationship is under strain. Yet the formal mechanisms designed to enhance autonomous decision-making such as living wills or advance directives, actually presuppose that the doctor-patient relationship is entirely satisfactory and based upon mutual trust and respect. The principle of respect for autonomy and the rule derived from it which requires informed consent serves as a corrective to paternalism and professional arrogance. But it involves a process of acquiring information (from the patient's perspective) and understanding the scope for decision (from the doctor's perspective) which includes continuous evaluation of the extent of freedom from coercion and manipulation. A patient can only express an autonomous choice in a trusting relationship. One can only act autonomously if one trusts that others can recognise what is autonomous and what can be overridden. For whilst autonomy must be respected it must also be reassessed. The fallacy of the market model lies in the belief that an autonomous choice can be expressed in a contract or document which can be substituted for the sensitive use of professional authority in a trusting relationship.

IX   Autonomy and Surrogacy

Introduction

Some of the confusions in the appeal to autonomous refusal are beginning to emerge. A serious problem concerns the employment of surrogates to express a patient's 'autonomous' choice. There are, for example, problems regarding who is an appropriate surrogate. Although it is accepted that surrogates should be close family members there are many who do not live in 'recognized' families, such as members of the gay community. There is also what Americans describe as 'the Florida syndrome', where elderly retired parents have lost contact with their offspring, although the latter may be called upon to make decisions without appreciating their parent's desires regarding therapy options. A similar problem occurs if it is the parent's in such circumstances who are called upon to make decisions on behalf of estranged offspring. This chapter will raise questions concerning extensions of the principle of autonomy to cover the appointment of surrogates. Should, for example, surrogates have the authority to override decisions made by a previously competent patient? It will be argued here that autonomous choice cannot be adequately represented in surrogacy arrangements and that the morally preferable course is a 'best interest' standard involving cooperation between surrogate and doctor.

Standards for Surrogate Decision Making

Some crucial distinctions need to be addressed when formulating guidelines for surrogate decision-making. One case involved a US court ruling concerning a severely mentally retarded cancer patient, Mr. John Storar with a mental age of 18 months who was 52 at the time of the proceedings, and whose mother's request for the discontinuation of blood-transfusions was turned down. (*Re John Storar*, 1981) Mr. Storar had never been competent. At the time of the proceedings he had been diagnosed as suffering from cancer of the bladder. Initially his mother, a 77-year-old widow, agreed to the recommended blood transfusions but then, after several weeks, she requested that they were discontinued. The Director of the Newark Development Center, where Mr. Storar was being treated, sought authorization to continue with the transfusions. Mrs. Storar cross-petitioned for an order prohibiting further transfusions. It was conceded that Mr. Storar found the transfusions disagreeable and was disturbed by the blood clots in his urine which followed the transfusions. He could not comprehend the purpose of the transfusions and on some occasions displayed resistance. There was also a body of medical opinion which asserted that the transfusions were merely prolonging a life of suffering. However, the Appeal Court refused his mother's request to abandon blood transfusions for his cancerous condition, setting limits to surrogacy stressing that no one, neither parent nor sibling, should decide that an incompetent should bleed to death. The basis of the court's decision was that because of Mr. Storar's retardation it was impossible to know what his wishes would have been before therapy for cancer was applied. 'The court's decision', says Zussman, (1992:175) 'involves an important legal principle. It distinguishes between formerly competent patients and never competent ones like Storar'.

In recent years US courts have operated with three distinct standards for surrogate decision making on behalf of incompetent patients. (Meisel, 1992) First, are subjective standards which require that the surrogate seeks to 'discover and effectuate the patient's own preferences expressed before the patient lost decision-making capacity'. (Meisel, 1992:342) This would involve attempts to discover the patient's known preferences and would rely on oral statements made by the patient before losing competence. The second set of standards are more hypothetical: they are the substituted judgements whereby the surrogate is required to 'make the best approximation of what the patient would or would not have wanted'. (*ibid*:342) Whilst the subjective standard asks 'what did the patient decide before losing decision-making capacity?' the substitute judgement standard asks 'What would the patient decide if the patient were able to decide?' In substitute tests the surrogate is obliged to consider the patient's value system for guidance in order to extrapolate what course of medical treatment the patient would choose, were he or she capable of choosing. Subjective and substitute tests, however, cannot be applied to patients who have been mentally incompetent from birth and hence have never been in a position to form views or hold and express values. The third standard is an appeal to the best interests of the patient, and is clearly unrelated to the principle of autonomy. For some commentators the 'best interest' test indicates a questionable distance from the principle of respect for autonomy, allowing others to make decisions regarding the quality of a patient's life. On the other hand 'best interests' and substitute judgement tests may coincide if the surrogate is committed to carrying out the known wishes of the patient. For this reason it is argued that the problem would be resolved if the law recognised a person's right to appoint a health-care agent in the event of a future incompetent state. Thus Ian Kennedy and Andrew Grubb (1994:1211) argue that, whilst in principle English law favours a 'best interests' test, in cases where the patient had previously been competent the courts could adopt the 'substituted judgement' test.

It is also questionable whether either the subjective standard or the substitute judgement standard can function as the autonomous preference of a patient no longer capable of decision-making. Kathryn A. Koch *et al* (1992) suggest that the belief that substitute judgement represents patient autonomy is a 'figment of our imagination' and argue that the best interest standard, based on an assessment of benefits and burdens, should prevail. Accordingly they maintain that there may be times, in the absence of any clear patient preference, when medical knowledge can re-assert itself against the wishes of a family, when the medical facts become so clear that decisions for level of care should rest with the doctors.

Subjective standards and substitute judgements have been rejected in English law which favours the 'best interest' test, where the medical carers of an incompetent patient make decisions in the patient's best interests in accordance with a responsible and competent body of relevant professional opinion. Serious doubts concerning the employment of surrogates to act on behalf of incompetent patients were expressed in the conclusion of the House of Lords Select Committee on Medical Ethics. (1994:55)

> ...the appointment of a surrogate to act for a patient who, through mental infirmity has never been competent to form a reasoned judgement, seems to stretch the concept of patient autonomy to breaking point. This would also be the case if the patient were a carefree young adult, living solely in the present, with no thought for the morrow and no true understanding that life may change for the worse, and having no taste or capacity for addressing the wider and deeper issues raised by grave illness, inability to communicate,

destruction of personal dignity and erosion of the quality of life.

The 'best interest' test, although perhaps better than subjective standards and substituted judgements insofar as it functions within the parameters of morally responsible professional standards, is not without problems. The term 'best interest', is employed in the English judicial system, and is used most successfully in determining the welfare of children in custody cases or the well-being of the mentally disabled where some kind of assessment or comparison is made between options and their likely outcome. A 'best interest' test is difficult to apply in decisions concerning the withholding or withdrawing life-prolonging therapy as it is impossible to make any meaningful comparison between continued life and the absence of it. A way forward might be to consider a distinction made by Ronald Dworkin (1995) between a patient's experiential interests and his critical interests. Most discussions concerning a patient's best interests refer to the actual experiential state of the person. But Dworkin suggests that there are other interests, critical interests, which are not experiential. These interests would encompass notions concerning the success of our whole lives of which the manner of our death is an important and integral aspect. Paying attention to one's critical interests may very well lead to a judgement, argues Dworkin, that it is in someone's best interests to opt for an early rather than a prolonged death. It might also be said, with reference to another person's critical interests, that an early death is not in one's best interests. Whilst this approach reveals the importance of relating one's whole life-project to the manner of death it is, perhaps, unhelpful when taking decisions in an ICU or in circumstances where the doctors and surrogates are not deeply involved in the patient's life.

Surrogate Decision Making and the Persistent Vegetative State

Respect for patient autonomy depends on a level of honest communication between doctor and patient. This is not an option for the neonate or severely brain damaged patient where arrangements for proxy or surrogate decision-making are frequently resorted to. This raises considerable ethical problems, particularly when decisions are made which involve the withdrawal of life-prolonging therapy. The limits to surrogate refusal were tested in the controversy surrounding the Cruzan case in 1990. Following a motor accident in 1983 Nancy Beth Cruzan remained in a persistent vegetative state. Convinced that there was no hope of recovery and that she would not have wished to go on living in that condition, Nancy's parents sought to withhold nutrition and hydration which was being artificially supplied through a tube. A court authorised removal but this was overruled, in November 1988, by the Missouri Supreme Court, which maintained that Nancy's parents could not exercise the right to refuse treatment on her behalf and that the state's unqualified interest in preserving life should prevail. The case was then taken up by the United States Supreme Court, on 25 June, 1990, which upheld the decision of the Missouri court by a 5 to 4 margin, finding that Nancy Cruzan had not made clear-cut expressions regarding her future incompetent state. It was not a matter that could be settled by appeal to autonomous patient choice. This ruling did not repudiate the rejection of medical attention by either a patient or a surrogate; it simply held that it was constitutional for a state to prevent the withdrawal of life-sustaining care 'in the absence of clear-cut instructions from the previously competent patient.' (Cantor, 1993:31) The Supreme Court did not impede the development of advance directives or the use of prior-designated surrogates; it simply insisted that such measures are adequately indicated by the previously competent patient.

One of the arguments advanced in support of the withdrawal of nutrition and hydration was the claim that prior to the accident she had made several remarks to the effect that she would not wish 'to face life as a vegetable' and that she believed that 'some conditions were worse than death'. Although she had not signed an advance directive it was argued that these prior statements amounted to an informed refusal. The court, however, did not accept this as sufficient evidence for an autonomous refusal. It should be stressed that the cost of life- prolonging therapy was not at issue in this case and there was no undue financial strain on the relatives. Nancy's daily food supply cost $7.80 and the cost of therapy was paid by the State of Missouri.

Yet those close to her maintained that her plight was intolerable. Several months after the case appeared before the Supreme Court a fresh hearing was held before the same county probate judge who had originally considered the case in order to hear new evidence of Nancy Cruzan's wishes. The court again ordered the removal of the feeding tube and in September of 1990 the State of Missouri withdrew its interest in prolonging her life. Shortly after her legally appointed guardian concurred with the family wishes and her feeding tubes were removed on 15 December, 1990 and despite an attempt by a group of protestors to enter her room and reconnect them, and six lawsuits and appeals from pro-life organizations, Nancy Beth Cruzan died on 26 December, 1990. Her death was reported in England, in *The Guardian* (27 December) in the context of a euthanasia decision. Under the heading 'Euthanasia woman dies' the report described how 'her parents satisfied the high court's euthanasia criteria.' The distinction between treatment abatement and euthanasia was apparently ignored.

It is, however, important to realise that diagnosis and confirmation of an irreversible persistent vegetative state precedes discussion about the termination of life-prolonging therapy, and that such diagnosis involves a lengthy procedure with built-in safeguards. In the guidelines for discontinuation of therapy for irreversible PVS patients the Medical Ethics Committee of the BMA (1992) outlined four safeguards. First, that every effort should be made at rehabilitation for at least six months after the initial injury; second, that diagnosis of an irreversible PVS should not be confirmed until at least 12 months after the injury; third the diagnosis should be confirmed by two other independent doctors, and fourth, that generally the wishes of the patient's immediate family will be given great weight, but that they should not be determinate.

There is an emerging consensus among medical experts that PVS patients should die. Cases have been cited of PVS patients being maintained alive purely for tax purposes and then having their life-sustaining therapy withdrawn in order to maximise insurance disability payments or pensions (Smith, 1988). In September, 1992, the Appleton International Conference, attended by specialists from nine countries, including the USA and Britain, brought out guidelines urging that PVS patients should be allowed to die. According to the Appleton Conference (1992:11)

> The patient who is reliably diagnosed as being in a PVS has no self-regarding interests. Consequently, unless a previously expressed advance directive requests it, there is no patient-based reason to continue life-sustaining treatments, including artificial hydration and nutrition. It is unkind to allow unrealistic optimism to be sustained and it is unfair to allow the prolonged consumption of societal resources in support of such patients beyond a period of education and adjustment for the family.

There are obvious problems with this statement. First, it is not clear that unrealistic optimism is either generated or sustained by life-prolongation. Second, there is a morally questionable link made between 'having no self-regarding interests' and 'societal resources'. Third, as pointed out in a dissenting note by some participants in the Appleton Conference, it is not obvious that 'having no self-regarding interests' rules out other moral interests, such as beliefs in the inherent value of life. It is not obviously unfair to maintain the life of a being that has no awareness of the quality of his or her life. The only reliable inference that can be drawn from a state of unawareness is that we do not know the value that person would place on the quality of life.

The arguments for and against unlimited life-prolongation for patients in irreversible persistent vegetative states will need to be addressed and, despite their poor quality of life, it must be said that no constitutional rights are violated by maintenance of therapy for such patients. There is, moreover, a societal interest in protecting the lives of PVS patients, who represent a paradigm case of dependent beings and we abandon that responsibility at the risk of damage to the structure of the human community. In a state beyond pain, unaware of her situation, Nancy Beth Cruzan could not be said to have been harmed by continuing medical treatment. She was certainly not in the same category as a pain-racked terminally ill cancer patient who has expressed an interest in foregoing further attempts at life-prolongation.

There is, however, serious concern over a tendency in cases like *Cruzan* and *Bland* to amalgamate surrogate decision-making with autonomous refusal of life-prolonging therapy. Nancy Beth Cruzan's wishes were not abundantly clear and if a surrogate had been appointed any decision made on her behalf would not have been her autonomous decision. It may be necessary in such cases to appoint a surrogate to act in a patient's best interests, with powers to refuse therapy. But the decision to authorise a surrogate cannot be based on an appeal to patient autonomy and self-determination. The introduction of a legal fiction that autonomous decisions can be made by others is incompatible with the principle of autonomy and could involve the re-introduction of paternalism as seen in the Netherlands where doctors have been known to make quality of life decisions without adequate consultation with their patients. Before long it could be claimed that the state provided the best mechanism for making autonomous decisions on behalf of its citizens. One starts with the requirement for surrogates that are familiar with the patient's known values, and proceeds to the point where the surrogates have but a limited knowledge of the patient's values, which then involves an appeal to what a reasonable person would choose, and ends with a position where the state, or its officials, exercise the choice. Such is the dialectic from libertarianism to authoritarianism.

Although close family members may be more familiar with the patient's views the possibility that the family may have interests which would not be of benefit to the patient sets limits on family proxy. A novel solution to this problem has been proposed by Linda L. Emanuel and Ezekiel J. Emanuel (1993) who argue that proxy decisions should be taken by communities of patients, and that health-care organizations be considered the unit of the community. There is considerable merit in this proposal as a community of patients, well-organized and in the possession of a collective history of similar cases, could make effective, sympathetic and informed decisions which would not be prejudiced by the professional interests of the hospital authorities on the one hand and the emotional turmoil within the family on the other hand. There is, however, still the possibility of tension if those acting on behalf of the community of patients were to directly oppose or override the known wishes of the family. But certainly arrangements whereby family members and the patient community could cooperate in reaching a joint decision would be advantageous. The Emanuels (1993:12) see recourse to communities of patients in terms of its 'usefulness in achieving patient autonomy'. This is an unfortunate way of presenting the case for more involvement with patient communities, as such procedures should not be seen as means of enhancing patient autonomy, but as means of reaching the right decision. What is missing in most of the surrogate decision arrangements is preservation of the patient's agency. This, by definition, is a problem if the patient is incompetent which is a state where the capacity for agency is lost. Autonomy cannot be surrogated and in certain circumstances we have to resort to the employment of mechanisms for making the *right* decision. Thus it may not be a question of obtaining an accurate account of the patient's wishes, but one of formulating the right decision.

Conclusion

Surrogate or proxy decisions are best resorted to but nevertheless limited to situations where decisions are required in the incompetent patient's best interests. It has been argued here that surrogacy arrangements do not derive their legitimacy from an extension of principles regarding autonomy. There are problems in determining whether proxies actually know what is in the patient's best interest.

Choices with regard to therapy abatement are not purely dependent upon the subjective deliberations of the rational individual, and are not reducible to the refusal of unwanted medical intervention. This is a myth that has been imported from questionable assumptions in political economy, and is of little benefit to medical practice and the sometimes agonizing decisions which have to be taken by patients and their relatives. Nevertheless, guidelines which foster greater autonomous choice should be informed by well-founded principles and beliefs that can stand the test of public scrutiny and debate, as well as the willingness of an informed public to apply them. Any changes to existing practices - and many are surely needed - should likewise meet similar tests.

An individual's right to therapy abatement can be protected from abuse in the context of a full understanding of autonomous choice; not merely the right to refuse but the opportunity to consider alternatives. Patient autonomy cannot be exercised abstractly; there are limits to autonomy which include the values upheld by professional carers. Limits are also required on the role of the surrogate in the refusal of therapy. Further safeguards should require that statutes giving legal power to advance directives are not framed in such a way that they can be later hijacked by euthanasia societies. It should not be forgotten that guards against the erosion of respect for life do not simply shore up religious beliefs; they provide protection to gravely ill and vulnerable patients. Policies endorsing therapy abatement and exercise of the right to forego life-sustaining therapy should carry cast iron guarantees that they will not be disadvantageous to the poor and undereducated members of society. It should also be recognised that advance directives may not turn out to be a satisfactory alternative to poor communication between doctor and patient and that their very success is dependent upon significant improvements in this relationship. It should also be noted that fears of unlimited life-prolongation could be greatly exaggerated. In an atmosphere of governmental indifference to the plight of the sick, with the notion of welfare tuned to market forces, there is a danger that self-determination can have a restricted meaning; the option of death in the context of an underfunded health service. This may not be the time to campaign for the right to refuse therapy, but rather the time to campaign for improvements to existing therapy.

Bibliography

Ackerman, F., 1991, 'The Significance of a Wish', *Hastings Center Report*, 21,4, July/Aug:27-29

Agich, G.J., 1990, 'Reassessing Autonomy in Long Term Care', *Hastings Center Report*, 20, 6:12-17

Airedale NHS Trust v Bland, [1993] 1 AII ER 821, 1993 12 BMLR 64 (HL)

Age Concern, The Centre of Medical Law and Ethics, Kings College, London, 1988, *The Living Will: Consent to Treatment at the End of Life*, London:Edward Arnold

Aldridge, Peter, 1994, 'Who Wants to Live Forever?', in *Death Rites*, eds. Robert Lee and Derek Morgan, London:Routledge, 11-36

Alpers, Ann, Lo, Bernard, 1992, 'Futility: Not Just a Medical Issue', *Law, Medicine and Health Care*, 20, 4:327-329

American Medical Association, 1986, *Current Opinions of the Council on Ethical and Medical Affairs*, 2, 18:12-13

American Medical Association, 1991, Council on Ethical and Judicial Affairs, 'Guidelines for the Appropriate Use of Do-Not-Resuscitate Orders', JAMA, 10 April, 265, 14:1868-1871

Anon, 1986, 'The Kings Peace', *The Times*, 28 Nov.

The Appleton International Conference, 1992, 'Developing Guidelines for decisions to forgo life-prolonging medical treatment', *Journal of Medical Ethics*, September, 18, Supplement

Battin, Margaret, Pabst, 1994, *Least Worse Death: Essays in Bioethics on the End of Life*, Oxford: Oxford University Press

Beach, Edwin, 1991 quoted in *Medical Ethics Advisor*, 7, 4, April:49

B.M.A., 1992, Sept., *Treatment of Patients in Persistent Vegetative State*, London:B.M.A.

Brennan, Troyen, A., 1992, 'Physicians and Futile Care: Using Ethics Committees to Slow the Momentum', *Law, Medicine and Health Care*, 20, 4:336-339

Brock, Dan, 1994, 'Advance Directives: What is it reasonable to expect from them?', *Journal of Clinical Ethics*, 5, 1:57-60

Brody, Howard, 1993, 'Causing, Intending and Assisting Death', *Journal of Clinical Ethics*, 4, 2, Summer:112-117

Buchanan, A., 1988, 'Advance Directives and the Personal Identity Problem', *Philosophy and Public Affairs*, 17, 4:277-302

Re. C., (A Minor) (Wardship: Medical Treatment) [1989] 2 All ER 782, CA

Re. C., 1993 NLJR 1642

Callaghan, Daniel, 1991, 'Medical Necessity, Medical Futility: The Problem-Without-A-Name, *Hastings Center Report*, 21, 4:30-35

Callaghan, Daniel, 1992, 'When Self-Determination Runs Amok', *Hastings Center Report*, March-April, 22, 2:52-55

Cantor, Norman, L., 1993, *Advance Directives and the Pursuit of Death With Dignity*, Bloomington and Indianapolis: Indiana University Press

Caplan, Arthur, L., 1992, *If I Were a Rich Man Could I Buy a Pancreas?*, Bloomington and Indianapolis: Indiana University Press

Capron, Alexander Morgan, 1991, 'In Re Helga Wanglie', *Hastings Center Report*, 21, 5:26-28

Capron, Alexander Morgan, 1995, 'Sledding in Oregon', *Hastings Center Report*:34-35

Childress, James F., 1990, 'The Place of Autonomy in Bioethics', *Hastings Center Report*, 21, 1:12-17

Clark, Angus, 1995, 'Medicine Cannot Serve Two Masters', in S. Bewley and R. Humphrey-Ward (eds), *Ethics in Obstetrics and Gynaecology*, London: RCOG Press:111-120

Cohen, Cynthia B., & Cohen, Peter J., 1992, 'Required Reconsideration of "Do Not Resuscitate" Orders in the Operating Room and Certain Other Treatment Settings', *Law, Medicine and Health Care*, 20, 4:354-363

Re. Conroy, In Re. Conroy, 98 N.J. 221, 486 A. 2d 1209, 1236, 1985

Cranford, Ronald E., 1991, 'Helga Wanglie's Ventilator', *Hastings Center Report*, 21, 4:23-24

Crawford, Ronald and Gostin, Lawrence, 1992, 'Futility: A Concept in Search of a Definition', *Law, Medicine and Health Care*, Winter, 20, 4:307-309

Van Delden Loes, J.M., and Van Der Maas, Paul J., 1993, 'The Remmelink Study: Two Years Later', *Hastings Center Report*, 23, 6:24-27

Dolley, Margaret, 1993, 'Public Uses Denmark's Living Will', *BMJ*, 306:414-5

Dunstan, Gordon, 1995, 'Should Philosophy and Medical Ethics be left to the Experts?', in Susan Bewley and R. Humphrey-Ward (eds), *Ethics in Obstetrics and Gynaecology*, London: RCOG Press:3-8

Dworkin, Ronald, 1995, *Life's Dominion*, London: Harper Collins

Emanuel, Linda L., and Emanuel, Ezekiel J., 1989, 'The Medical Directive: A New Comprehensive Care Document', *JAMA*, 261:3288-93

Emanuel, Linda L., and Emanuel, Ezekiel J., 1989, 'Does the DNR Order Need Life Sustaining Intervention?, *The American Journal of Medicine*, 86:87-90

Emanuel, Linda L., and Emanuel, Ezekiel J., 1993, 'Decisions at the End of Life: Guided by Communities of Patients', *Hastings Center Report*, 23, 5:6-13

English, Dan C., 1994, *Bioethics: A Clinical Guide For Medical Students*, London: Norton Medical Books

Fenigsen, Richard, 1989, 'A Case Against Dutch Euthanasia', *Hastings Center Report* 19, 1:22-30

Fenton, Julie, 1994, 'Caring for Patients who cannot or will not eat' in Geoffey Hunt, ed., *Ethical Issues in Nursing*, London: Routledge:72-89

Fried, Terri; Stein, Michael D.; O'Sullivan, Patricia S.; Brock, Dan W., and Novack, Dennis H., 1993, 'Limits of Patient Autonomy', *Archives of Internal Medicine*, 153:722-728

Fung, K.K., 1993 'Dying For Money: Overcoming Moral Hazard in Terminal Illness Through Compensated Physician-Assisted Death', *American Journal of Economics and Sociology*, 52, 3:275-288

Gorman, J.L., 1987, 'Philosophical Competence', in *Moral Philosophy and Contemporary Problems*, ed., J.D.G. Evans, Cambridge: CUP:71-80

Gorowitz, Samuel, 1993, *Drawing The Line: Life, Death and Ethical Choices In An American Hospital*, Philadelphia: Temple University Press

Gostin, Lawrence O., 1993, 'Drawing a Line between killing and letting die: the law, and law reform, on medically assisted dying' *The Journal of Law, Medicine and Ethics*, 21, 1:94-101

Grant, Edward R., 1992, 'Medical Futility: Legal and Ethical Aspects', *Law, Medicine and Health Care*, 20, 4:330-335

Hastings Center, 1987, *Guidelines on the Termination of Life Sustaining Treatment and Care of the Dying*, Bloomington: Indiana University Press

Henk, A.M.J. ten Have, and Jos V.M. Welie, 1992, 'Euthanasia: Normal Medical Practice', *Hastings Center Report*, 22, 2:34-38

High, Dallas M., 1993, 'Advance Directives and the Elderly: A Study of

Intervention Strategies to Increase Use', *Gerontologist*, 34:342-349

Holm, Soren, 1994, 'My (Danish) Living Will', *Hastings Center Report*, 24, 1:2

Hope, Tony; Sringings, David, and Crisp, Roger, 1993, 'Not Clinically Indicated: Patients' interests or resource allocation?' *BMJ*, 306:379-381

House of Lord Select Committee on Medical Ethics, 1994, *Report of the Select Committee on Medical Ethics*, Volume I, Session 1993-94, House of Lords, London: HMSO

Hunt, Geoffrey, 1994, *Ethical Issues in Nursing*, London: Routledge

Baby J, 1990, *Re. J* (A Minor) (Wardship: Medical Treatment) [1990] 3 AII ER 930, [1991] Fam 33 (CA)

Kapp, Marshall B., 1994, 'Futile Medical Treatment: a review of the ethical arguments and legal holdings', *Journal of General Internal Medicine*, 9 March:170-177

Keene, Barry, 1978, 'The Natural Death Act: A Well-Baby Check-Up on its First Birthday', *New York Academy of Sciences*, 315:344-355

Kennedy, Ian, 1988, *Treat Me Right*, Oxford: Clarendon

Kennedy, Ian and Grubb, Andrew, 1994, *Medical Law, Text and Materials*, 2nd Edition, London: Butterworths

Keown, John, 1992, 'On Regulating Death', *Hastings Center Report*, 22, 2:39-43

Koch, Kathryn A.; Meyers, Bruce W., and Sandroni, Stephen, 1992, 'Analysis of Power in Medical Decision-Making: An Argument for Physician Autonomy', *Law, Medicine & Health Care*, 20, 4:320-325

Kouwenhoven, W.B.; Jude, J.R., and Knickerbocker, G.C., 1960, 'Closed-Chest Cardiac Massage', *JAMA*, 173:1064-1067

Kutner, Luis, 1969, ' Due Process of Euthanasia: The Living Will, A Proposal', *The Indiana Law Journal* 44:529-554

Lamb, D., 1985, *Death, Brain Death and Ethics*, London: Routledge

Lamb, D., 1987, *Down the Slippery Slope: Arguing In Applied Ethics*, London: Routledge

Lamb, D., 1992, 'Death and Personal Identity', *Trivium*, 27, *Death and the Value of Life*: 43-56

Law Commission of England and Wales, 1993, The Law Commission Consultation Paper No. 129, *Mentally Incapacitated Adults and Decision-Making: Medical Treatment and Research*, London: HMSO, 29

Longmore, Paul K., 1987, 'Elizabeth Bouvia, Assisted Suicide and Social Prejudice', *Issues in Law & Medicine*, 3, 2:141-168

Longmore, Paul K., 1987,a, 'Whose Life is this Anyway?', in Sam

Maddox ed., *Spinal Network*, Colorado: Spinal Network and Sam Maddox

Lynn, Joanne and Teno, Joan M., 1993, 'After The Patient's Self-Determination Act: The Need for Empirical Research on Formal Advance Directives', *Hastings Center Report*, 23, 1:20-24

Meisel, Alan, 1992, 'A Retrospective on Cruzan', *Law, Medicine & Health Care*, 20, 4:340-353

Morris, Jenny, 1993, *Pride Against Prejudice*, London: Women's Press

Maclean, Anne, 1993, *The Elimination of Morality*, London: Routledge

New York Public Health Law, 1987, Code 2961. 9

Nolan, Kathleen, 1987, 'In Death's Shadow: The Meaning of Withholding Resuscitation', *Hastings Center Report*, 17, 5:9-14

Nowak, Rachel, 1992, 'The Dutch Way of Death', *New Scientist*, 20 June:28-20

O'Connor, John J. Cardinal, 1989, *Catholic New York*, 20 July

Pearlman, Robert Allan, 1994, 'Are We Asking the Right Questions?' *Hastings Center Report*, Special Supplement, 24, 6:24-27

Pellegrino, D., 1992, 'Doctors must not Kill', *The Journal of Clinical Ethics* 3:95-102

Rachels, James, 1986, *The End of Life*, Oxford: OUP

Rawls, John, 1971, *A Theory of Justice*, Cambridge Mass: Harvard University Press

Remmelink Committee, 1991, Paul J. van der Maas *et al*, 'Euthanasia and other Medical Decisions Concerning the End of Life', *Lancet* 338, 14 Sept: 669-74, *Commissie Onderzock Medische Praktijk inaake euthanasie, Medische Beslissingen het Levenseinde*, The Hague: SDU Uitgeverij, 1991

R V Bodkin Adams ([1957] Crim. L.R. 365)

Sacred Congregation of the Doctrine of the Faith, 1980, Declaration on Euthanasia, cited in the *Report of the Select Committee on Medical Ethics*, 1984

Rie, Michael A., 1991, 'The Limits of A Wish', *Hastings Center Report*, 21, 4:24-27

Robertson, John A., 1991, 'Second Thoughts on Living Wills', *Hastings Center Report*, 21, 6:6-9

Sachs, Greg A., 1994, 'Increasing the Prevalance of Health Care Planning', *Hastings Center Report* Special Supplement, 24, 6:13-16

Saunders, John, 1994, 'Medical Futility: CPR', in *Death Rites* eds. Robert Lee and Derek Morgan, London: Routledge:72-90

Schneiderman, L.J.; Pearlman, R.A.; Kaplan, R.M., and Teetzel H., 1993, 'Do Physicians own preferences for life-sustaining treatment influence their perception of patient's preference?', *Journal of Clinical Ethics*, 4:28-33

Sedler, Robert A., 1993, 'The Constitution and Hastening of Inevitable Death', *Hastings Center Report*, 23, 5:20-25

Silverman, Henry J.; Fry, Sara T.; and Armistead, Niti, 1994, 'Nurses perspectives on implementation of the patient self-determination act', *The Journal of Clinical Ethics*, 5:30-38

Scofield, Giles A., 1991, 'Is Consent Useful When Resuscitation Isn't?', *Hastings Center Report*, 21, 6:28-36

Singer, P., and Kuhse, H., 1985, *Should the Baby Live?*, Oxford: O.U.P.

Smith, David, 1988, 'Legal Issues Leading to the Notion of Neocortical Death', in R.M. Zaner, ed., *Death: Beyond Whole Brain Criteria*, Dordrecht: Kluwer:111-114

Soloman, M.Z., 1991, *Life and Death Decisions: Physicians Perspectives and Their Implications for Professional Education*, Ann Arbor: University of Michigan

Soloman, M.Z., 1992, 'Futility as a Criterion of Limiting Treatment', Letter, *New England Journal of Medicine*, 327, 7:1239

Spooner, Jeffrey M., 1994, 'Dying Under The Maple Leaves', *Hastings Center Report*, 24, 4:2

Re John Storar, 1981, 420 WE 2d 64 (NY CA)

Re T (adult: refusal of treatment) [1992] 4 AII ER 649, (1992) 9 BMLR 46 (CA)

Templeton, Allan, 1995, 'Informed Consent', in Susan Bewley and R. Humphrey Ward (eds) *Ethics in Obstetrics and Gynaecology*, London: RCOG Press:287-297

Teno, Joan M.; Nelson, Hilde Lindemann, and Lynn, Joanne, 1994, 'Advance Care Planning: Priorities for Ethical and Empirical Research', *Hastings Center Report*, Special Supplement, 24, 6:32-36

Teno, Joan M.; Lynn, Joanne; Phillips, Russell S.; Murphy, Donald; Youngner, Stuart J.; Bellamy, Paul; Connors, Alfred F. Jr.; Desbiens, Norman A.; Fulkerson, William and Kraus, William A., 1994, 'Do Formal Advance Directives Affect Resuscitation Decisions and the Use of Resources for Seriously Ill Patients?' *The Journal of Clinical Ethics*, 5, 1:23-37

Tomlinson, Tom, and Brody, Howard, 1990, 'Futility and the Ethics of Resuscitation', *JAMA*, 264, 10:1276-80

Twycross, Robert G., and Lack, Sylvia A., 1986, *System Control in Far Advanced Cancer: Alimentary Symptoms*', London: Pitman

Veatch, Robert M., 1993, 'Foregoing Life-Sustaining Treatment: Limits to the Consensus', *Kennedy Institute of Ethics Journal*, 3, 1:1-19

Virmani, Jaya; Schneiderman, Lawrence, J., and Kaplan, Robert M., 1994, 'Relationship of Advance Directives to Physician-Patient Communication', *Archives of Internal Medicine*, 154:909-913

Re: Helga Wanglie, 1990, No. PX-91-283, Fourth Judicial District (Dist. Ct. Probate Ct. Div.) Hennepin County, M.N.

Wells, Celia, 1994, 'Patients, Consent and Criminal Law', *The Journal of Social Welfare and Family Law*, 1:65-78

Weir, Robert F., 1990, *Abating Treatment With Critically Ill Patients: Ethical and Legal Limits to the Medical Prolongation of Life*, Oxford: O.U.P.

Youngner, Stuart J., 1987, 'Do Not Resuscitate Orders: No Longer Secret But Still A Problem', *Hastings Center Report*, 17, 1:24-33

Zussman, Robert, 1992, *Intensive Care: Medical Ethics and The Medical Profession*, Chicago: Chicago University Press

Index

Acts and Omissions 3, 4, 19, 25-33, 97
Agich, G.J. 118-119
Airedale NHS Trust v Bland 23, 29, 93, 95-100, 134
Alpers, A. 88
Alzheimer's disease 122-3
Andrews, K. 98-99, 109
Appleton Conference 77, 115-116, 133-134
Aristotle 11

Baby C. 21-22
Baby J. 21
Battin, M.P. 36-37, 108
Beach, E. 116
Bergsted, K. 120
best interests 130, 131, 134-135
Bingham, Sir Thomas 80, 93
Bouvia, E. 116-118, 122
Bosely, S. 119
Botros, S. 97-98
Brennan, T.A. 88
Brennan, W. 92-93
British Geriatrics Soceity 30, 32
BMA 32, 47-48, 97, 133
Brock, D.W. 46-47
Brody, H. 27-28, 78-79, 83-85
Brown, J.M. 9
Brown, Sir Stephen 95-96
Bush, G 17

Callaghan, D. 28, 75
Cantor, N.L. 43, 45, 47, 49, 52, 58-60, 87, 123-126, 132
Caplan, A. 5-7
Capron, A.M. 55, 78
Carvel, J. 33
Clarke, A. 109
Childress, J.F. 125
Christian Medical Fellowship 19, 53
Clarke, A. 109
Cohen, C.B. 66, 69-70
Cohen, P.J. 66, 69-70
Conroy, C. 39, 92
Crawford, R. 81
Crisp, R. 106
Cruzan, N.B. 92-93, 131-134

Delden, van 34, 37
Dellaportas, G. 104
Descartes, R. 11
Devlin, Lord 31, 32
disability 56-60
Dolly, M. 40
Donaldson, Lord 22, 23, 120
Dunstan, G. 10
Dutch Physician's League 35
Dworkin, R. 131

Emmanuel, E.J. 44, 121, 135
Emmanuel, L.L. 44, 121, 135

ENABLE 57
engineering ethics 5-9, 15
English, D. 63
euthansia 14, 17-37, 40, 42,
  51-61, 70, 71, 79, 87, 94,
  96-97, 102, 106, 114-116,
  133, 136
EXIT 41

Fenigsen, R. 33
Fenton, J. 94-95
Flynn, E. 51
Frenchay Health-care NHS
  Trust v S 93
Fried, T. 115
Fung, K.K. 102-104

Gaff, Lord 23, 99
Gorman, J.L. 11
Gorowitz, S. 110
Gostin, L.O. 26, 87
Grant, E.R. 79, 80
Green, A. 98
Grubb, A. 130

Have, ten, AMJ. 36
High, D.M. 49
Holm, S. 40-41
Hope, T. 106

House of Lords Select Committee
  on Medical Ethics 19, 24,
  30, 32, 35, 41, 42, 44, 52,
  53, 57, 97, 110, 130, 131
Hunt, G. 9
hydration and nutrition 86,
  91-100, 133-134

Information technology 110-111
Intensive care 66, 69, 72, 73, 81,
  131

Kant, I. 11
Kapp, M.B. 75, 82
Kaplan, R.M. 45
Kendall, M. 119
Kennedy, I. 20, 21, 42-43, 130
Keown, J. 33-35
Kevorkian, J. 26, 30
Koch, K.A. 130
Kuhse, H. 20
Kutner, L. 51-52

Lack, S. 20
Laws, Justice 80
living wills (advance directives)
  3, 14, 18, 24, 33, 38-61,
  70-71, 87, 91, 97, 112,
  121-127, 132, 136
Lo, B. 88
Longmore, P.K. 56-58, 117-118
Lynn, J. 44, 50

Maas, van der 34
McAfee, L.J. 121-122
Maclean, A. 1, 2
McLeod, B 98
Meisel, A. 129
moral agency 10, 12, 15, 74, 76,
  82, 86, 88, 89, 91
Morris, J. 56-57

Nelson, H.L. 50
Nolan, K. 65

O'Connor, J.J. 25

paternalism 56, 63, 82-84,
  112-114, 118, 126, 134;
  limited paternalism 15, 65,
  73-74, 89, 101
Paterson, S. 98
Pearlman, R.A. 50
Pellegrino, E.D. 27

persistent vegetative state 39, 54, 74, 76, 81, 85, 86, 92-96, 98-100, 109, 110, 131-135
personhood 4, 5
Plato 10, 11
positivism 6, 7, 75
President's Commission 68-72

quality of life 131, 134
Quinlan, K 39, 79

Rachels, J. 29
rationing 81, 82, 101-110
Rawls, J. 113
Re C. 23
Remmelink Report 33-36
Re T. 22-23
Robertson, J.F. 43-44, 122
Rodriguez, S. 26

Sachs, G.A. 50
Saunders, J 63, 72-73, 89
sanctity of life 12
Schneiderman, L.J. 45-46
Scofield, G. 75, 105
Sedler, R.A. 30
Silverman, H.J. 45
Sinjer, P. 20
Smith, D. 133
Socrates 2
Soloman, M.Z. 83
Springings, D. 106
Storar, J. 128-9
suicide 26, 27, 30-32, 52, 56-58, 70-79, 87, 97, 102, 114, 116-117
SUPPORT 46

Taylor, Lord 21
Templeton, A. 49
Teno, J.M. 44-46, 50
Terence Higgins Trust 41

Tomlinson, T. 83-85
Twycross, R. 20

utilitarianism 1, 6, 47, 80

Veatch, R.M. 93-94
ventilation 26, 31-32, 72, 85-87, 121
Virmani, J. 45-46

Wanglie, H. 80, 85-87, 89
Weir, R.F. 18, 24, 51
Welie, J.W.M. 36
Wittgenstein, L. 1

Youngner, S.J. 62, 68

Zussman, R. 3, 66, 113, 129